Woman Far Walking

Woman Far Walking

Witi Ihimaera

HUIA

First published in 2000 by Huia Publishers,
39 Pipitea Street, P O Box 17-335,
Wellington, Aotearoa New Zealand.

ISBN 1-877241-51-2

Text © Witi Ihimaera
This edition © Huia Publishers

Cover photograph: Ross T. Smith, from the Hokianga series, 1997-98.
Designed, typeset and printed in Aotearoa New Zealand.

All applications to:
Playmarket
PO Box 9767
Wellington, New Zealand
ph 64-4-382 8462

With grateful thanks to all Māori women for their strength, wisdom, passion and leadership.

Contents

Introduction

This script is the revised fifth draft of *Woman Far Walking*. It was specifically written for publication by Huia Publishers and therefore may differ in some details to the performances during the play's first run during the International Festival of the Arts, Wellington, March 2000. This fifth publication draft takes into account the revisions and suggestions which arose from the workshop on the play which was held in the English Department's Drama Theatre, University of Auckland, 6–8 December, 1999. My thanks are due to those present at the workshop: Carla van Zon, director, New Zealand International Festival of the Arts; Hone Kouka, director, Taki Rua Theatre; Cathy Downes, director of *Woman Far Walking*; Rachel House, actor; Rima Te Wiata, actor; Diane Prince, designer; Mark McEntyre, designer; Murray Edmond, dramaturg; Mei-Lin Hansen, colleague of the English Department; and Jenny Gibbs. Thanks also to my parents, Tom and Julia, whose story this is. As always, my love to Jessica Kiri and Olivia Ata, my constant inspiration.

Woman Far Walking is a play about a woman who, in the year 2000, is 160 years old. People know her as Tiri Mahana but her real Māori name is Tiriti o Waitangi Mahana and she was born on 6 February 1840. As she herself says, 'When I was a little girl I always looked forward to meeting the person

I had been named after. It was a shock when I discovered that my namesake was not a person but a piece of paper, the Treaty of Waitangi.'

The outer structure of *Woman Far Walking* is provided by Tiri Mahana's 160th birthday party. Throughout the day we get to know important occurrences in Tiri's life and history. The day comes to a climax with the arrival of the governor-general with a telegram from the Queen.

The inner structure of the play takes place inside Tiri's memory and her dream world. Within this world, five incidents form a recurrent motif. The first incident occurs in childhood when, as a six-year-old girl, she is told by her mother to go with two weavers to cook for them: she is always waiting for her mother to come to take her home and, in the end, at the age of thirteen runs away. The second incident is when she is forty-two and a member of Te Kooti's rebellious army fighting the Pākehā in 1888; she survives the Ngatapa killings. The third incident is the flu epidemic, 1918, when she is seventy-eight, the only elderly woman to survive and to look after four remaining children of her tribe. 'Why me?' she asks. The fourth incident is the Springbok Tour, 1981, when she is 141 years old. The fifth incident occurs in 1990 when her beloved valley – the place where she was taken by the weavers and which was left to her in their will – is subject to land development. Tiri stands in the path of the earth-moving equipment. As the play progresses all the strands of past and present begin to intertwine. 'Sometimes,' Tiri says,

> the memories flow like a river. The currents cross and re-cross and, when the passions are in full flood, they join, swollen, together. You live this long, these things happen. Reality and unreality. Yesterday and today. Madness and sanity. One minute there. Next minute gone. But *you*

> still live on and all that life, that history, is like waves of
> the sea bursting above you, curling you down into the
> sand –

The themes of *Woman Far Walking* involve the survival, struggles and resilience of the Māori people, as shown through the life of one woman. In her lifetime Tiri has had to bury two husbands and all her children – except one son. It is from that son, Pirimia, the only one of her children to survive the flu epidemic, that the larger Mahana clan has grown. However, there is a secret attached to Pirimia, which we only discover at the denouement of the play.

Woman Far Walking is also a play of humour: when Tiri is forty, she is visited by Death and she tells him, 'Come back in thirty years.' When Death finally comes for her in the last pages of the play she asks, 'What took you so long! Did you forget?' As well, *Woman Far Walking* is a play about parental love. All her life, Tiri has been waiting for her mother to come and get her and take her home. As she dies, she seems to see her mother and she regresses into childhood: 'Have you come to get me, Mum? Is it time to go home now?'

Woman Far Walking is for two actors. One actor plays Tiri as a 160-year-old woman, sitting in a wheelchair but, from time to time, able to get up and walk with the aid of callipers or two walking sticks. The other actor is Tilly, in her mid-30s, a guest at Tiri's wedding, constantly interrogating Tiri's version of events. Tilly has a congruence with Tiri but often exhibits a critical role which sees both characters argue and pull against each other, and sometimes do battle with each other. Both Tiri and Tilly are in conversation about Tiri's life and history. They should be played by two actors who have some physical resemblance to each other. They share certain gestures and other characteristics in common, such as a certain quivering hand movement or way of standing at emotional moments which indicates defiance. Depending on their understanding of kawa, the actors may further inflect the text with personal cultural utterance and action as appropriate to their interpretation.

The play is for two actors, and is written to be accompanied by a mix of audio, stage and lighting effects conveying the events of Tiri's history and her life in the present day. The set is minimal and as indicated in the playscript.

Woman Far Walking plays for ninety minutes with an interval after the first two acts.

The haka 'Ka Panapana' was composed by Ngāti Porou relatives of Moana Ngarimu to acknowledge that the warrior spirit also involved women. Other waiata, details and expressions used in the play are also contemporary. As I have mentioned earlier Tiri's memories flow like a river. The currents cross and re-cross and, often, Tiri pulls things from the past into the present and takes things from the present and puts them in the past. This is how it is with memory. The events of Tiri's life are therefore more appropriately seen as happening in a continuum in which past and present exist as one and at the same time in a single continuous dramatic reality.

Witi Ihimaera
March 2000

First Performance

Woman Far Walking was originally commissioned by New Zealand Festival 2000 and the first performance was co-produced with Taki Rua Productions at Te Papa Soundings Theatre, 17 March 2000.

> *Director –*
>   Cathy Downes
>
> *Set and Costume Design –*
>   Mark McEntyre and
>   Diane Prince
>
> *Lighting Design –*
>   Jo Kilgour
>
> *Music composed by* Gareth Farr
>
> *Sound Design –*
>   Matt D'Herville
>
> *Kaiako Haka me te Waiata –*
>   Tere Harrison
>
> *Rākau Tapu –*
>   Tuari Dawson

Cast

Te Tiriti o Waitangi Mahana, 'Tiri' –
Rachel House

Tilly –
Rima Te Wiata

Crew

Production manager –
Robyn Tearle

Stage manager –
Cathy Knowsley

Assistant stage manager –
Marlena Campbell

Cast

TE TIRITI O WAITANGI MAHANA
Also known as Tiri, born on 6 February 1840, the year of the signing of the Treaty of Waitangi between Māori and Pākehā.

TILLY
A young woman in her mid-thirties.

Other characters appear as voices from TIRI'*s past and present. They accompany the stage action.*

The Present

FRED
Tiri's great-great-great-great-grandson, fifty-four years old, Māori.

JESSICA
Tiri's favorite mokopuna, ten years old, Fred's daughter, of Māori and Pākehā descent.

ANGELA
  Fred's wife and Jessica's mother, Pākehā.

REPORTER
  Male, in his late twenties, Pākehā.

GOVERNOR-GENERAL

The Past

TE KOOTI WARRIORS

SETTLERS

NGATAPA WARRIORS

FIRING SQUAD AND DRUMMER

FIRST WORLD WAR SOLDIERS

FIRST WORLD WAR CITIZENS

ANTI-SPRINGBOK PROTESTERS

SMALL POLICE SQUAD

DAME KIRI TE KANAWA

FOUR PĀKEHĀ SOLDIERS

Prologue

The stage is bare and dark. Head bowed, in a wheelchair, is an old woman, TIRI. She is dressed in a white nightdress. Her hair is white, waist length, and she wears it swept from the back of her neck and falling over one shoulder across her front. She has her walking sticks in both hands.

A sound like a gourd being shaken.

TIRI lifts her head and leans forward. The spotlight is merciless, showing her wrinkles, white hair and all the signs of extreme old age. She gathers the audience into her gaze.

TIRI: I am 160 years old. I was born on 6 February, 1840. I am an aberration. A freak. People make the sign of the cross when they see me because I am against Nature, an affront to God; they think Dracula must have bit me on the neck and made me into one of the living dead. Well if he did, he was the one who died.

My whakapapa, my genealogy, takes me back to the people of Te Tai Rawhiti, the East Coast. I grew up at a time when the iwi Māori ruled the land. In those days before jet planes my ancestor, Paikea, came to these islands riding a majestic whale. The sky was a man and the earth was a woman — and I still greet them both —

Ihia te rangi! Ihia te mana!
Ko Ranginui kei runga,
ko Papatuanuku kei raro,
tēnā kōrua, tēnā kōrua, tēnā kōrua.

My mountain has always been Hikurangi, the first place in the world to greet the sun. When I was young I loved to watch the sun rising above the sea and to feel the earth quickening around me. There have been too many suns on too many mornings. That red ball, ascending from the morning sea, only tires me now.

Then one day, long before I was born, a visitor came to our islands. Hairy. White as a ghost. Smelling different. My grandmother was there. It was 1769 and she saw a huge, frightening, white-winged bird coming across the water into Tolaga Bay. She said that Captain Cook alighted from the bird and his sailors looked like goblins. They had eyes in the backs of their heads because they rowed their boats sitting with their backs to the land. They had three legs, and the third leg was called a musket. My grandmother told me that they welcomed this new goblin but — he killed them with his musket. Ever since, I have been at war with him.

Turuki turuki, paneke paneke!
Turuki turuki, paneke paneke!
Tēnei te tangata pūhuruhuru
Nāna i tiki mai whiti te rā!
A hupane, a kaupane!
A hupane kaupane whiti te rā!

TIRI *pauses, then talks directly to a member of the audience.*

You want to know what a dinosaur looks like? Look at me. I'm a T-Rex. No comet, no Noah's flood, no volcanic eruption, has finished me off. I'm still here. Like you, I had a mother whom I adored and a father whom I loved. I was not always — like this. People tell me I don't look my age — what do you think? They say I only look 130! Back then the blood danced young in my veins and everybody said I was beautiful like my mother.

I loved my mother. All she had to do was tell me what she wanted and I would do it. She would call, 'E Tiri! E Tiri! Haramai! Haramai koe!' and I would go to her. 'Do this, Tiri,' and I would do it. I was obedient to her because I loved her. I loved her so much that I kept watch on her all night. I would crawl into bed with her. I was afraid that she might not be there when I woke up. And I'd hold her tight, to make sure she'd be there at daybreak. My ten-year-old mokopuna, Jessica, she does the same thing with me now. But it's me who doesn't want to let her go! There's nothing like holding the future in your arms.

I have lived longer than my mother, my sisters and brothers. I have outlived their children and their children's children and their children's children's children. I have survived my first husband, my second husband and all the loved companions of my youth. The young always think only they enjoy the embrace of a husband. When they look at me they cannot believe a woman of my age has ever known passion. But I have known such beautiful husbands, such sweet men. They will always be young to me. I would not want them to see me as I am now. They are gone — and all the beautiful babies we made, they too are gone, gone, gone.

Oh, my plump, beautiful babies ...

TIRI *bends and clasps her abdomen, remembering the babies that have come from her womb. She begins to sing a waiata tangi. As she sings, she is accompanied by the sound of waves crashing on a beach.*

Rimurimu, tere tere, ki te moana e!
Tere ana ki te ripo i waho e!
Tirohia atu ki waho rā, marino ana e!
Kei roto i ahau, marangai ana e —

TILLY *appears at a 'doorway' at the back of the stage, directly behind* TIRI. *She is youthful, beautiful, dressed for a party and seems to come unwrapping herself from dreams. She stands immobile, listening to* TIRI'S *singing. All of a sudden* TIRI *can't go on. She begins to weep, clutching her abdomen tighter as if in absolute pain.* TILLY *replicates the motion, keeping it still for a moment. She continues* TIRI'S *song for her.*

TILLY: Seaweed drifting, drifting, drifting,
Carrying my children away from me.
Drifting, floating, floating, drifting,
Toward the whirlpool on the sea.
Look out further, all is calm there
But my heart rains with stormy tears,
Seaweed drifting, floating, drifting,
My children floating away on the sea —

TIRI: Kei te tio te huka, i runga o ngā hiwi!
Kei te moe koromeke te wairua e!
Rite tonu tō hanga ki te tīrairaka e!
Waihoki tō hanga, te wairangi e ...

As she sings, TILLY *makes appropriate actions with her hands. Slowly she approaches* TIRI *and stands behind her. Together,* TIRI *and* TILLY *sing the rest of the waiata in unison, harmony and counterpoint, building it to an emotional climax. By the end of the waiata their actions are exactly similar.*

TIRI/TILLY: Rimurimu, tere tere, ki te moana e!
Tere ana ki te ripo i waho e!
Tirohia atu ki waho rā, marino ana e!
Kei roto i ahau, marangai ana e —
Kei te tio te huka, i runga o ngā hiwi!
Kei te moe koromeke te wairua e!
Rite tonu tō hanga ki te tīrairaka e!
Waihoki tō hanga, te wairangi e ...

A flute takes up the melody and seems to float the tune into the auditorium. TIRI *and* TILLY *listen and watch until the flute's notes fade. Then* TIRI *stiffens as she realises* TILLY *is there.*

TIRI: Not you again.

TILLY (*trying to humour* TIRI): As long as you're around, I'm around. You know I always come on your birthday.

TIRI: Always uninvited. Why don't you go away and leave me alone?

TIRI includes the audience in her anger. She propels her wheelchair around the stage.

TIRI (*to audience*): All of you, go away. Just because I've lived longer than anyone does that make me a freak? A side-show exhibit? Left high and dry like a waka in a museum where there are no seas? Or stuffed and put into a glass case like a huia with glass eyes and plastic bones wired together? Is this all I am to anyone?

TIRI *is too late.*

TILLY *(starts to karanga)*: Haere mai rā i te reo o te rā, haere mai rā
　　Haere mai rā e kui mā, e koro mā i te pō
　　E tama mā, i te karanga o tō tātou tipuna
　　Haere mai rā ...

TIRI *looks at* TILLY *and the audience. Her voice becomes hostile, a warning.*

TIRI *(to audience)*: So. You're staying with me then. Ka pai. To war, to war? Don't say that I have not given you due warning.

TIRI *stamps her walking sticks on the floor. It is like an announcement. She stamps them again, repeatedly. Then stops.*

Act One

Scene One

The lighting flickers, as if people are throwing shadows as they approach. The soundtrack echoes with giggles and hushed noises. The voices and noises are invasive, hissing all around the theatre.

TV REPORTER (*V/O*): Sir, shouldn't we knock?

FRED (*V/O*): Nah! If she's not up by now, she should be. Are you awake, Kui?
    It's time for you to face the cameras! Are they rolling, boys? Get away from the door, Jessica.

JESSICA (*V/O*): But Daddy, my nanny will still be asleep.

> *The theatre reverberates with* FRED's *knocking. On stage,* TIRI *and* TILLY *put their hands to their ears.*

FRED (*V/O*): Are you there old lady?

ANGELA (*V/O*): Oh Fred! Where else would she be! Jessica, didn't you hear daddy? Get away from the door.

CHORUS (*V/O*): Surprise! Happy Birthday! Happy Birthday! Happy Birthday!

JESSICA (*V/O*): This wasn't my idea, Nani. All of you, leave my nani alone.

> *On stage, TIRI and TILLY are fearful of the invasive shadows. The theatre fills with the sound of clapping. At the sound TILLY starts and tries to hide.*

REPORTER (*V/O*): Happy birthday, Mrs Mahana. Tell us, what is it like to be the oldest woman in the Commonwealth? What is it like to be the oldest woman in the world?

> *Flashbulbs pop, heightening the sense of disorientation. TIRI begins to strike out with one of her walking sticks. There is an echo effect on the REPORTER's words which fade into silence.*

Scene Two

Onstage, TIRI is striking out with one of her walking sticks. She tires. TILLY comes forward and laughs nervously. TIRI points one of her walking sticks at TILLY.

TIRI: Auē, te mahi o te Pākehā! And what are you laughing at?

TILLY: I was enjoying what you were doing. You're still able to surprise me, even after all these years.

TIRI: Don't you get smart with me, girl. Such a stupid, stupid question. And only my moko, Jessica, to protect me against everybody. How do I feel? When you're young you have all the time in the world to love, to live, to love again, and the air is so sweet to breathe. You get older, Time starts to go faster and everybody starts to die on you. First you feel lucky, so lucky that you're still here and cheating Death! Then you realise the air is no longer sweet. It stinks of the dead and they've all gone, your generation. The next generation comes and then it too is gone. And the next. And the one after that and they keep on piling up the dead the dead the dead —

> TIRI *is spiralling downward, her mouth opening and closing as if she is gasping for air.* TILLY *quickly diverts her attention.*

TILLY: So what have you been telling everybody about yourself? (*Mischievously*) Have you told them how you got your name?

TIRI: No.

TILLY: You mean, you haven't introduced yourself yet? (TILLY *steps forward and faces the audience.*) Her father was Rangiora Te Teira and her mother was Turitumanareti Matete. There were eleven in the family. (*To* TIRI) You were the fourth girl, eh? You lived at Puketewai, just out of Tolaga.

TIRI: How do you know all this? Who told you? Yes, that's right! That's right!
I was named Tiri for short, and as I was growing up I thought my longer name came from one of my aunties. I always looked forward to meeting my auntie and I used to ask —

TILLY: Can I go to see Auntie Tiri?

TIRI: It wasn't until I was six, all grown up, that one of my
brothers said to me – Hey! Did you fullas know you were
named after the Treaty of Waitangi?

> TILLY *laughs.*

It was no laughing matter, girl. It was a shock to know
that Auntie Tiri was a piece of paper. And what a namesake. A fraud. Full of lies and Pākehā promises. How
would you like to carry the name of the document which
took Māori land?

TILLY: You always wanted to spit on the Treaty didn't you!

TIRI: Āe, but to do so would have been to spit on my own
name and I couldn't do that.

TILLY: But you had a good childhood, didn't you Tiri, with
your iwi, your whānau, your family, Mum and Dad. Then
one day –

TIRI: Hei aha –

> *It is too late.* TILLY *hums to herself and kicks off her
> shoes. She advances to centre stage and takes the stance of
> the women's haka.* TIRI *whimpers, then straightens up.*

TILLY: My mother was teaching me how to do the women's
haka.

TIRI: Hope!

> TILLY *puts her hands on her hips. She is bashful, and*
> TIRI *smiles and remonstrates with her.*

TIRI: Auē, e hine. How you going to learn, daughter, if you don't pay attention. Hope!

> TILLY *does the movement properly this time.* TIRI *nods, satisfied. She calls out again.*

TIRI: Ringa whiua! Ararā! Ka panapana!

> TIRI *leads 'Ka Panapana', a women's haka, a leitmotif throughout the play. The performance is underpinned with a rhythmic bass beat, like the thud of stamping feet. As the haka continues,* TIRI *tutors and corrects* TILLY's *mistakes.*

TILLY: I a ha ha auē!

TIRI: Ka rekareka tonu taku ngākau ki ngā mana ririki pōhatu whakapiri

TILLY: Kia haere mai!

TIRI: Te takitini

TILLY: Kia haere mai!

TIRI: Te takimano kia pare tai tokotia ki Aotearoa!

TIRI/TILLY: Hi ha auē!

TIRI: He mamae, he mamae!

TIRI/TILLY: I a ha ha auē!

TILLY: Ka haere, ka haere taku pōhiri ki te tai whakarunga!

TIRI/TILLY: Hoki mai, hoki mai taku tinana!

TILLY: Ka haere, ka haere taku pōhiri ki te tai whakararo!

TIRI/TILLY: Hoki mai, hoki mai taku tinana!

TIRI: Kia huri au ki te tai whakatū a Kupe ki te tai o
  Matawhero i motu mai!

TIRI/TILLY: E ko hoariri ki roto i aku ringa kūtia rawatia kia
  pari tōna ihu!
  Hi, ha, auē!

> *At the end of the haka* TILLY *looks proudly at* TIRI – *but*
> TIRI *is overcome with memories.*

TIRI: E Mā! E Mā! (*To* TILLY, *but motioning to the audience*) I don't
  want to tell them. You tell them.

TILLY: I was playing with my brothers and sisters and
  showing my mother how I could do the women's haka.
  My mother was praising me and telling me how good I
  was when, all of a sudden, two women and an elderly
  man came riding out of the sun.

> TILLY *shades her eyes and then looks at* TIRI.

TILLY: Who are these people, Mum?

TIRI: E Tiri, me haere koe.

TILLY: You want me to go with them?

TIRI: Yes, darling. They are weavers and, because you are my
  fourth daughter, they have asked if they can have you.
  Their work is very sacred and they are not allowed to
  touch food. They need someone to cook for them.

TILLY: Okay.

TIRI: Look after them and be obedient.

TILLY: Āe, e Mā. (*To audience*) Straight away I jumped up on the horse behind one of the old women. Just like that. In the clothes I was wearing. No shoes. No sentimental goodbyes. No saying 'E noho rā' to the rest of the family. All I took with me were the instructions from Mum.

TIRI: You have to be the keeper of the fire. Look after the old ladies, keep their fire alight, do your best and go.

TILLY: I loved my mother and did everything my mother told me to do. When she said, Go, I went.

TIRI (*in a girl's voice*): Yes! Up! Onto the horse and off and away!

TILLY: Gee, those old people lived a long way away. In a valley, four days ride to get there, near the sea where there were no roads. The brother was mentally retarded and they looked after him. Their house was a small whare, and way over the other side of the paddock was the kāuta, the kitchen, separated from the sacred work of the weaving.

TIRI (*in a girl's voice*): Oh, I remember those cloaks, those korowai! They were all colours, reds, yellows, purples, greens, blues, like all the rainbows of the world were being born there. In that old house. Far at the end of the world.

TILLY (*to audience*): As soon as I arrived, I was treated as an adult. No excuses for being six. I was put straight to work and, because my mother had told me to be obedient, I did the work without complaint. I was shown the place where I was to sleep — on the floor at the foot of the bed of the senior woman. I slept there for seven years. Every morning the kuia and the old man all woke up to say karakia, prayers.

TIRI (*in a girl's voice*): Oh, those old hīmene! They wove magic all around that old house. They called the rainbows over the valleys, through the mist and into the sacred work so that the aho tapu, the sacred thread, would be in the weft of the weave!

TILLY: Straight after the karakia I would run barefoot in all weather to the old kāuta. (*Miming, hands on hips, shaking her head*) Look at this place! Rain coming through the roof. Window broken. Gee, who was the last cook here? You sure are a broken-down old kāuta! Okay, let's patch up the roof first, so that the rain won't go spit, spit, spit and try to spit the fire out. And now, are you still alive, fire, where I buried you in the ashes last night? There you are! (*Mimes uncovering the embers and blowing on them*) Come on, fire, start to smoke! Here's some twigs to help you! Come alight now! Yay! (*Looks at the audience self-importantly*) Not bad, eh!

TIRI: All that cooking, day and night. This was my responsibility because if there was no fire there was no cooked breakfast. After a while I never ever had to use a match! But the first months, though, I got a lot of punishment for my mistakes. I suppose those old ladies wanted me to learn faster.

> TILLY *is humming and mimes putting big iron pots onto hooks above an open fire and brushing the smoke away from her eyes.*

TILLY: Fire's going good now! Where's my bucket? Now down to the stream to get some water. Gosh this bucket's heavy. Hey! I'll make a sled out of two planks of wood! And a harness for myself so I can pull the sled to the stream and back.

TIRI: Yes, that's right, that's right! That's what I did! After a while, though, I had a brainwave. The old people had a pet dog and I looked at him.

TILLY: Hmm ... (*Whistling, as if to a dog*) Kia ora, kurī! Come here, boy. How are you today? Good boy. Good boy. You may be old but you can still do valuable work, eh, kurī? Can you take this rope in your teeth and pull the sled down to the stream? You can? Good dog. Good boy.

TIRI (*looking on as* TILLY *mimes patting the dog*): That old dog, he became my best friend and we loved one another very much. Every day me and him would take the water back to the kāuta, where I would fill the pots and bring the water to the boil.

TILLY: All this before it was dawn, eh. All this, every morning, for seven years.

> TILLY *mimes stoking the fire. She brushes her forehead and sits patiently waiting for the water to boil. She takes a piece of string from a pocket of her dress and begins to make cat's cradle patterns. Meanwhile,* TIRI *is humming a waiata tawhito.*

TILLY: So what shall I make us for dinner today, eh kurī? Eels or dried shark meat?

TIRI: The senior of the women showed me how to catch eels —

TILLY: Only one time — and then I had to do it by myself from then on.

TIRI: No excuses.

TILLY: No 'Can you show me again?'

TIRI: Just the once.

TILLY: I would gather worms or nice juicy huhu grubs and thread them on to a whītau, a flax thread. Then (*Whistling to her dog*), Come on, kurī! Help me drag this old tin basin down to the river.

TIRI: There I would sit, dangling the whītau into the water, waiting for the eels to bite.

TILLY: Come on, Mister Tuna ...

> TILLY *mimes fishing with a line.* TIRI *comes beside her and looks down, as if at water, pointing out eels.*

TILLY (*whispering*): Here's one coming!

TIRI: I would see them, gliding greyly, sliding like sinister dreams up to the surface of the water.

TILLY: Haere mai, tuna! Come and get a nice, fat, juicy worm! Gotcha!

TIRI: Once the eel swallowed the worm it wouldn't let go and —

TILLY: Flick! Quick, here comes another one!

> TIRI *and* TILLY *duplicate the action of hooking the eels.*

TIRI: I would pull the eel out and into the basin. And —

TILLY: Flick! Another eel! Flick, another. Flick, and another.

TIRI: In all that time, my dog would sit silent because the dog he knew that his life, and those of the old people, depended on my fishing skills, eh boy!

TILLY: Good boy! Good dog!

> TILLY *stands up, mimes putting the harness on her dog and whistles to the dog to pull the basin to the kāuta. She takes her string out again and holds the pattern up to the sky.*

TILLY (*to dog*): Look, kurī! I can bring the rainbow down from the sky and trap it in my string!

TIRI (*to audience*): But catching the eels that was easy. What was hard was when people brought us shark meat.

TILLY: How I hate curing and drying this meat. It makes my hands raw.

TIRI: The people were generous in those days. They sometimes brought a bag of flour in exchange for the cloaks and woven mats the weavers made.

TILLY (*to audience*): The old ladies would give the flour to me and say —

TIRI: E Tiri, mahia mai he parāoa.

TILLY: You want me to make a Māori bread? Okay. (*To audience*) The old people never had butter with their bread. But as a special treat they would sometimes get some dripping for me. They told me they had grown to love me because I was obedient and did my work well. Very soon, I had all the household tasks well under control. For seven years I did this, and I was growing all the time in places that I never dreamed of!

TIRI: But my one dress began falling apart so I decided I'd better learn how to weave so I could make a new one. I asked the senior kuia to show me.

TILLY (*miming*): E Kui, will you teach me how to weave so I can make me a dress?

TIRI: No, Tiri, your job is to keep the fire alight.

TILLY: I felt very sorry for myself and was embarrassed because my body was showing through my dress. My mother had always told me I should be modest — and whenever visitors came I began to hide because I was so ashamed that I didn't have a nice dress. Then one night the two kuia surprised me. They said —

TIRI: This is for you, Tiri.

> TIRI *has a simple cloak which she gives to* TILLY.

TILLY: This cloak for me? It's so soft on my shoulders! And look, when I move it is full of rainbows!

> TILLY *dances around* TIRI *with delight. She mimes taking the cloak down to the stream and trying to look at herself in the water.*

TIRI: But I was not happy there. All those years I was always wondering when my mother would come to get me.

TILLY: I loved my mother. All she had to do was to tell me something and I would do it. I was obedient to her. But, as time went by I'd go up to the road with my dog and wait and wait and wait. (*Miming*) E kurī, can you see her? Is she coming? Is that her? Is it? And I rehearsed every day what I would say to her when she arrived. Have you come to get me, Mum? Is it time to go home now?

> TIRI *and* TILLY *mime together looking up and down a long road. Looking up and down. Up and down.*

TILLY (*mimes throwing a stone*): She isn't coming.

TIRI: No, not today. Perhaps tomorrow.

TILLY: We'd better get back to the kāuta. Come on, dog.

TIRI: Well, one year passed and then another. Sometimes the old people got sick. I was sent out to gather herbs to make them better. I lived an isolated life, knowing only those old people — nobody else, just them.

TILLY: Me and my pet dog began to do more and more heavy work. I loved that old dog. I depended on him. He was obedient to me. But one day, when we were returning with water from the spring, he stopped. I whistled for him (*Whistles*) but he began to pant in a strange way. He lay down. When I saw that my dog was going to die, I got so wild that I picked up a stick and started to beat the dog, trying to make it stand up.

TIRI (*while TILLY is beating her dog*): E tū, e kurī. Haria atu te wai ki te kāuta! Get up, dog. We have to take the water back to the kāuta!

TILLY: But my poor dog just couldn't do it. Quietly he began to whimper, almost as if he was asking my forgiveness for leaving me to do all the work. Then he died. Just like that. No excuses. One minute there, next minute gone. Don't leave me alone, kurī, don't leave me to do all the work by myself. I cried, of course, though I knew it was a sign of weakness. When my dog died I didn't want to go on by myself.

TIRI: Blowing on the fire every morning.

TILLY: Covering the fire every night.

TIRI: Cooking. Sleeping on the dirt floor. Waiting.

TILLY: Some people say I ran away but I didn't really. I just left. I wanted to be with my mother.

TIRI: When I got home I saw my sisters and brothers and I ran up to them —

TILLY: Kia ora! Hello! It's me!

TIRI: But I'd been away for so long that they didn't recognise me. 'We thought you were dead!'

TILLY: Where's Mum? Why hasn't she come to get me?

TIRI: Kua mate kē a Māmā.

TILLY: She's dead?

TIRI: She passed away five years ago.

TILLY: So that's why she didn't come for me. But you would have come, eh Mum. If you had been alive you would have come, eh. You wouldn't have left me there. You wouldn't.

Scene Three

TIRI *begins to weep.* TILLY *unwraps herself from the memory. Her face is impassive as she looks at* TIRI.

TILLY: Crocodile tears —

TIRI: Who are you! Why are you always here? Why are you making me remember —

TILLY (*flaring*): Because you only tell some of the story, not all of the story. You did wrong, Tiri, wrong.

TIRI: You don't know anything.

TILLY: After you found out your mother was dead you know you should have gone back to those old people.

TIRI: I wanted to stay in Puketewai. I wanted to grow up with my brothers and sisters.

TILLY: You were supposed to be the keeper of the fire, you know what Mum said —

TIRI: I wanted to be with my people, with people my own age —

TILLY: Oh, why bother to pretend, girl?

> TILLY *puts her shoes back on. She looks up and down, as if along a long road. She pretends that some young man is coming. She smooths down her dress in a provocative manner. She gives a wolf whistle and pretends she has a stone in one of her shoes.*

TIRI (*to audience*): Yes, all right! That's what really happened. My first husband, Tamihana, came into my life. I was thirteen and he was fifteen — and he knew a ripe apple when he saw one.

TILLY: Oh such a strong handsome boy. We saw each other and were struck by lightning.

TIRI: Ha! Lust more like it.

TILLY: Why do you have to be so cynical? Just because you're old, all dried up and your womb shrivelled to nothing, don't try to pretend that you don't remember the innocence, the sweetness of your first husband. The touch of a man's skin, no, nobody forgets that. How soft and frightening. The feel of him as you receive him into you. The way he cries out and spills into you his seeds of life — there was no going back, after that, to a valley where rainbows were called to come every morning. So don't try to make out that there was some other high and mighty reason why you didn't go back to those old weavers. Tell the truth —

TIRI: And nothing but? All right. I became pregnant, is that what you want me to tell them? Does that make you feel better?

TILLY: Yeah, you fell for that old cock-and-bull story that if you did it standing up —

TIRI: Don't you belittle me! My first-born is not to be belittled. What mother does not remember the carrying of a child inside her, the belly like a melon ripening to split —

TILLY: Not being able to see your feet for months —

TIRI: When the labour pains began, the midwife was called —

> *A full moon rises. Silhouetted,* TIRI *and* TILLY *enact the birth of* TIRI's *first-born.* TIRI *chants an oriori.*

TIRI (*to* TILLY): Push, girl! Here it comes!

TILLY: Auē te mamae!

TIRI: Haramai e tama ki te ao o Tane!
Haumi e! Hui e! Taiki e!

> *Onstage,* TIRI *enacts holding up the baby and cutting its birth cord. On the soundtrack the sound of a smack and a baby crying. The moon fades away.*

TIRI: My first child, a son was born, in 1854. I called him Tamihana after his father. Then came three more, one for every year, Hiria, Ruka and Kereopa. I was healthy and my womb was fertile.

TILLY: And Tamihana, well, he was *too* healthy! Always wanting to be inside me.

TIRI: They didn't have football or television in those days —

TILLY: Before I knew it, I had another son — Moanaroa — and the year was 1860 and I was twenty years old and —

> TILLY *clasps herself and shivers. She sees that* TIRI *has also sensed something is approaching. The lights begin to flicker light and shadow and, on the soundtrack, comes a sound like a bulldozer mixed in with the other sounds symbolising the history that Pākehā settlement has brought with it.* TILLY *begins to retreat but* TIRI *goes forward to confront the sound.*

TIRI: It is true, he does look like a goblin.

TILLY: Look! His complexion as pale as the moon and just as still and silent.

TIRI: Is that the scent of his spoor? Sour and bitter?

TILLY: And is that his helpmate, his goblin woman, floating across the earth on a black cloud? Let's hide away, they are looking at us and their eyes are blue like a devil's. Did you ever see such eyes, Tiri?

TIRI: And is this their mark? This toeless imprint, these sprays of urine over the land?

TILLY: And, look! More pale people, coming down the road. Settlers. Pale faces. Putting up fences. Pale riders upon pale horses. Towns sprouting up all around us. Pale, pale, faces. Replacing our godsticks with their surveyor's pegs.

TIRI: To war! To war!

> TILLY *begins to chant the words, 'Turuki, turuki, paneke, paneke.'*

TIRI/TILLY: Turuki, turuki, paneke paneke —

> *The two women continue to chant the words over and over again. As they do so, the words are taken up by a chorus on the soundtrack. The chorus is accompanied by a rhythmic bass beat.* TIRI *and* TILLY *slowly back away. The chant increases volume and becomes a crescendo.*

CHORUS (V/O): Tēnei te tangata pūhuruhuru
    Nāna i tiki mai whiti te rā!
    A hupane, a kaupane!
    A hupane, kaupane, whiti te rā —

> *The haka creates a bridge from Act One into Act Two.*

Act Two

Scene One

TIRI *and* TILLY *retire to the 'doorway' position on the set. The action is continuous as the haka repeats itself and ceiling-to-floor ropes are added to the set.*

TILLY helps TIRI into a brown russet coat, buttoned up to the neck. TILLY herself changes into the kind of clothes that guerilla Māori fighters wore during the New Zealand Wars.

The action is still continuous as the lighting changes to flickering shadows. On the soundtrack, hissing around the theatre, we hear the voices of the DIRECTOR and the REPORTER.

DIRECTOR (*V/O*): Right-o, kid. Ready to go?

REPORTER (*V/O, nervously*): Yes, I think so.

DIRECTOR (*V/O*): We want you to interview the little girlie first —

TIRI: Who are they talking about!

TILLY: Jessica.

TIRI: She'll give them their beans!

While the interview continues, TILLY *walks swiftly through the set, securing the ropes to the floor and testing them. She begins to put bandoliers of ammunition on* TIRI *and herself.*

DIRECTOR (*V/O*): Give this all the energy you've got. The whole world wants footage of the old girl's birthday. The BBC. CNN. *Oprah* is featuring the story tonight — the oldest woman in the world. They want history. They want blood and guts. They want sensation. And they want it all in three minutes! So go for the jugular. Quiet on the set. (*A clapper board signals the cue.*) And action!

REPORTER (*V/O, to* JESSICA): Your parents have told us that you are the favorite of all Mrs Mahana's grandchildren.

JESSICA (*V/O*): I'm not a grandchild exactly. I'm one of her mokopuna. And I'm not a little girlie either.

TILLY (*laughing*): That's telling them! Go for it, Jess!

REPORTER (*V/O*): Could you explain for our American audience what mokopuna means?

JESSICA (*V/O*): I'm one of her descendants. There are over a thousand of us now.

REPORTER (*V/O*): A thousand? Wow. And is it true that once upon a time Mrs Mahana was a queen of the cannibals?

TIRI: Yes, and you better watch out, I still eat people!

JESSICA (*V/O, and glaring*): That was one of the names you all called her. It stuck

REPORTER (*V/O*): But the Māoris were cannibals, weren't they? Weren't they? And did your grandmother ever tell you about the wars, the Māori Wars?

> *At the* REPORTER's *final words* TIRI *gives a quick nod to* TILLY *to come to her side. As* TILLY *does so, at the run, she picks up a musket with shoulder sling and throws it to* TIRI. TIRI *puts the musket across her shoulder.*

> *Suddenly the soundtrack booms and roars with the sounds of battle. The stage lights flash and flicker, simulating the battle. Musket shots, bugle calls signal the attack.*

Scene Two

The battle simulation ends.

TIRI (*in karanga*): Ko te tangata he toa, ko te wahine he toa. (*Speaking*) The man is a warrior, so too is the woman a warrior. And when we go into battle, *all* of us go. Not just the men by themselves. The women and children too. If you are ever against us don't spare the women or the brats that we have because in war, gender and age make no difference. We are soldiers all. Famed for our ferocity. Where you see one woman you see — a thousand. The fight is not over until *we* are dead.

> TIRI *makes a sign and* TILLY *takes up her peruperu staff. Slowly and ritually, executing fighting movements with the staff,* TILLY *approaches the audience in the wero. At the end of the wero she becomes still.*

With a tremendous intake of breath, she stands on her walking sticks. She too approaches the audience, her walking sticks thudding on the floor of the stage.

TILLY: Te mātauranga a te Pākehā he mea whakatō mō wai rā, mō Hātana! Mō Hātana, I tell you! Do you hear me? Do you hear!

TIRI begins to shout out a peruperu drill sequence. At every order TIRI takes the appropriate position, jabbing and probing with her staff against an invisible opponent. As happened during the 'Ka Panapana' women's haka sequence, TIRI's instructions are first admonitory and then approving.

TIRI (*enigmatic, referring to* TILLY's *drill*): You should have finished me, way back then, when you had the chance. So, my eternal shadow, are we ready?

TILLY (*to audience*): When the wars began they were called the Māori Wars, then the Land Wars and then the New Zealand Wars.

TIRI: Nobody asked us what we called them — the Pākehā wars. They were fought in the Waikato, the Taranaki, the King Country, the north. Then they came to the East Coast, twenty years after they had begun.

TILLY: Tamihana heard that the prophet Te Kooti had escaped from the Chathams and was returning to Aotearoa.

TIRI: The prophet is calling for followers. We must go.

TILLY: The children too?

TIRI: Yes.

TILLY: No good standing around wasting time. Let's go.

> TIRI *and* TILLY *load their muskets and enact a rifle practice.*

TILLY (*to audience*): Whareongaonga, 10 July 1868. Word had come that Te Kooti had escaped his wrongful imprisonment on the Chathams, seized a boat, and arrived home. We went down to the beach to help him and the 297 who had come with him.

TIRI (*singing a prayer*): Let my people go, Pharaoh, let us be freed from the slavery of Egypt. Let us journey to our promised land of Canaan.

TILLY: As soon as I saw the Kooti I knew he was a prophet of God and that I would follow him to the ends of the earth.

TIRI/TILLY (*making the sign of the upraised hand*): Korōria ki Tō Ingoa Tapu.

TILLY: But the cohorts of Pharaoh arrived. Major Biggs and eighty militia.

> TIRI *and* TILLY *stand back to back, sighting their muskets into the air and circling.*

TILLY: Throw down your guns and surrender.

TIRI: E hoa, Biggs, let us go, let us go in peace unto our own land of Canaan.

TILLY: Instead, Biggs fell upon us with his goblin horde. Repeatedly he tried to stop us as we pilgrimaged to the Ureweras. He attacked us with 140 soldiers at Paparatu. He attacked us again at Te Koneke. As we traversed the

Ruakituri, Biggs tried to stop us there also — this time with 236 men.

TIRI: The Lord was with us and He turned the weather against Biggs.

TILLY: But in all the attacks by Biggs many of our followers were killed. So it was that the prophet hardened his heart and sent a message to Biggs at the military garrison at Matawhero.

> *On the soundtrack, the conch or the braying of a pūtātara. Tongues of flame shoot up around the set.*

TIRI (*in a trance*): Three times, Biggs, you have attacked me and three times I have asked you to leave us alone. You still pursue us in our pilgrimage. Therefore I shall take my people up unto Puketapu Mountain. There I will establish my church, the Ringatū. And from there, in November, I shall fight you. This is my declaration of war for, verily, I see that you will not relent and you will not let my Israelites out of their bondage unto Egypt.

> *The horns blows again. TIRI sings in religious fervour. The horns repeat themselves like echoes over the following exchange.*

TIRI: E te Atua, show us the way to face this net of death, and take us up to Thee so that we may glorify Thy Holy Name.

TILLY: And we thrived on Puketapu Mountain. And many came to join us. When November came we took our utu.

TIRI/TILLY: Korōria ki Tō Ingoa Tapu.

TILLY looks at TIRI and gives her a swift nod. The horns die away.

TILLY: Te Kooti asked me to be one of his lieutenants.

TIRI: Not Tamihana — me.

TILLY: He saw that I was good at battle and fearless in the kill.

TIRI: Will you be my left hand of God, with which I might smite the Egyptians?

TILLY: Yes.

TIRI: Tamihana was with the wing of raiders comprising the prophet's right hand of God. We kissed each other, kissed our children and then departed Puketapu Mountain.

The following sequence is continuous. Over it the horns bray repeatedly like hunting horns.

TILLY: Monday 9 November, 6.30 PM. I led my squad of men on the run towards Matawhero. We went by way of the Ngatapa Valley, past Repongaere Lake. There we waited. Under cover. One minute to midnight —

TIRI: Attack —

TIRI/TILLY: Korōria ki Tō Ingoa Tapu.

TILLY (*interjecting commands as if to her followers*): Kia kūtia! Au! Au! Whiti! Whiti e! Close your ranks! Cross over!

TILLY looks at the audience.

TIRI: You remember Matawhero, don't you?

A drum is added to the soundtrack. Its beat is slow and irregular at first but, as the sequence proceeds it increases – together with the horns – in both volume and speed. The soundtrack introduces the amplified noises of whirring wings, flax rustling, men and women breathing heavily.
TIRI *and* TILLY *performed movements choreographed to simulate a guerilla Māori attack.*

TIRI: Kia wherahia! Au! Au! Whiti! Whiti e!
    Open your ranks! Open them! Cross over!

TILLY: Nekeneke! Nekeneke! Nekeneke!

TIRI: Ka tiritiria! Ka tiritiria! Au! Au!
    Scatter! Scatter!

TILLY: A tama tū! A tama tū! Au! Au!
    Stand your places! Stand your places!

TIRI: Whano! Whano! Au! Au!
    Go! Go!

TILLY: Hui e! Taiki e! Au! Au!
    Gather! Fight!

TIRI/TILLY: Au! Au!

The sequence reaches a climax with TIRI *and* TILLY *firing their muskets into the air, reloading and firing. The physical action on the stage is amplified by the soundtrack which now includes loud rifle shots and screams and horses whinnying, receding into fade-out.*
On stage, TIRI *is in a trance.*

TIRI: Biggs, my old enemy, my nemesis.

> *On the soundtrack, the horns are braying, loudly at first and then receding into silence. The tongues of flames go down and the dawn comes up.*

TILLY: 10 November 1868. The dawn rose at 4.45 AM. The retaliation was to all intents and purposes over.

TIRI (*whispering, peering at the audience*): Huihuingia mai rā o tātou mate. Huihuingia. Gather our dead. Take them with us.

TIRI/TILLY: Korōria ki Tō Ingoa Tapu.

Scene Three

A sudden flare and the lighting returns to the white of daylight.

TILLY: They say we massacred sixty-three people.

TIRI: Did we? It was a military attack. War is war.

TILLY: They say that some of the victims were in the church praying when we slaughtered them.

TIRI: Were they? I can't remember a church and people praying. By that time we were on the run from Pharaoh's cohorts. We should have known that Pharaoh would want *his* own revenge, *his* own utu, for what we had done. He pursued us, oh how his soldiers pursued us, and in the pursuit many fell. My eldest girl, Hiria, she was reloading my musket —

TILLY: Here we are, Matua —

TIRI: She was smiling, handing the musket to me, when a bullet smashed through her brain. No time to say goodbye. One of my sons, which one was it?

TILLY: Kereopa —

TIRI: He was seven, I think. He fell way back as we ran but I had to look after my squad so I pushed him into the flax and told him I would come back for him.

TILLY: Ka kite anō, Matua —

TIRI: When I went back to find him —

TILLY: My body was floating in a stream, slit from throat to stomach. Friendly Māoris, fighting on the government side, had scalped me. Five pounds per scalp.

TIRI (*in a wild passion, singing*): E te Atua, homai te aroha ki a mātou mate, kua hoki atu rātou ki a koe e ... O Lord, give your love to the souls who return to you e ...

TILLY (*to audience*): Christmas, 1868. Our clifftop fortress, Ngatapa. That's where Pharaoh cornered us. Let me show you. Down there was Pharaoh with seven hundred troops. He built a series of forts coming up the ridge, closer and closer. Up here, at Ngatapa, this is where we made our stand. We were running out of ammunition and out of water and food.

Pharaoh couldn't get us out.

TIRI: Then on the ninth day —

> *The soundtrack booms with mortar fire coming from afar, whistling overhead and seeming to come into the theatre with repeated explosions.*

TIRI: Death rained down upon us and 125 were struck down. I lost my eldest son and I myself was wounded. I went to the prophet.

TILLY: If we all stay here, we shall all surely die. Let me continue to be your left hand of God. Escape with Tamihana, your right hand, and let me remain with the weak and the wounded to delay Pharaoh.

TIRI: Te Kooti did not want to do this. I reminded him —

TILLY: Ko te tangata he toa, ko te wahine he toa.

TIRI: The back of the pā was a steep cliff leading down into forest below. On the evening of 4 January 1869 we women made flax ladders for the prophet and all the able-bodied followers, to escape. Tamihana was weeping.

TILLY: Go, husband and take our remaining children, Ruka and Moanaroa, with you.

TIRI: By the splintered moon I watched them leave.

TILLY (*singing*): Let our people go, Pharaoh, let us be freed from the slavery of Egypt. Let us journey to our promised land of Canaan.

TIRI/TILLY: Korōria ki Tō Ingoa Tapu.

> *The wind starts to howl. A bullroarer increases the tension.* TIRI *and* TILLY *advance to the very apron of the stage, as close to the audience as they can get.*

TIRI (*to audience*): It is 5 January 1869. Your Pākehā soldiers took our fortress this morning. They found only the wounded, fourteen men, sixty-six women, the rest children.

TILLY: We should have known that you would have no mercy. Kill us if you will but know this, Pharaoh, after us will come others. Ka whawhai tonu mātou, ake, ake, ake!

> *On the soundtrack, cries of terror.* TIRI *and* TILLY *mime being pushed further forward toward the audience as if it was a cliff.*

TIRI: Oh Lord, we taste soon the bitter taste of Death. We ascend to you by the whirlwind path of Enoch. Korōria ki Tō Ingoa Tapu.

TILLY: The wind howls with the voices of spirits. The sky is red and bloodied with the dawn of a day that none of us will live to see. We shall be cut down in the flowering of our years.

TIRI: Auē, the children cut down, cut down too. We will sing the songs of Jehovah. We will hold each other in companionship so that we all go together into the next world.

TILLY (*miming to a soldier*): Hey, Pākehā! One last puff of your pipe, eh? The tobacco is so sweet! Hey, tell your companions to give the children quick deaths so that they will not feel pain, eh?

> *A kettle drum begins its drumroll.*

TIRI (*raising a fist to the audience*): Let our people go, Pharaoh, let them be free from the slavery of Egypt. Oh Lord, let us depart the grace of this world. Glory be to Your Holy Name.

TILLY (*miming*): Listen, everybody. Come, haramai, come nearer to the cliff so that when we are shot we shall fall over the cliff, eh? Let us not give Pharaoh the pleasure of more of our scalps, eh?

SOLDIER (*V/O*): Muskets at the ready!

TILLY: Oh the air is so cold, so wonderful to breathe!

> *The soundtrack cries of terror reach a climax. The cries stop as* TIRI *uses her walking sticks to come forward. She stamps them on the floor.* TILLY *joins her. They look back, calling to their companions to join them on the edge of the stage. Near the very end of the soundtrack sequence the voices are amplified and sound like the shrill barking of a pack of dogs.*

TIRI/TILLY: Kia kaha! Kia manawanui! E tū! E tū! Nekeneke! Nekeneke! Tama tū tama ora! Wahine tū wahine ora! Tamariki tū tamariki ora! Au! Au! Au! Au!

SOLDIER (*V/O*): Aim!

> *Defiantly* TIRI *and* TILLY *reprise 'Ka Panapana'. On the soundtrack the chorus joins in.*

TIRI/TILLY: Ararā ka panapana!

ALL (*V/O*): I a ha ha auē!

TIRI/TILLY: Ka rekareka tonu taku ngākau ki ngā mana ririki
pōhatu whakapiri
Kia haere mai!
Te takitini!

Kia haere mai!
Te takimano kia pare tai tokotia ki Aotearoa e!

ALL (*V/O*): Hi ha auē!

TIRI/TILLY: He mamae, he mamae!

ALL (*V/O*): I a ha ha auē!

TIRI/TILLY: Ka haere, ka haere taku pōhiri ki te tai
        whakarunga!

ALL (*V/O*): Hoki mai, hoki mai taku tinana!

TIRI/TILLY: Ka haere, ka haere taku pōhiri ki te tai
        whakararo!

ALL (*V/O*): Hoki mai, hoki mai taku tīnana!
        Kia huri au ki te tai whakatū a Kupe ki te tai o
        Matawhero i motu mai!
        E ko hoariri ki roto i aku ringa kūtia rawatia kia pari
        tōna ihu
        Hi, ha, auē!

The haka reaches a climax. The kettledrum is at its peak.

SOLDIER (*V/O*): Fire!

*The rifles volley again and again, shredding the haka at
each volley, echoing away into silence.*

TILLY: I remember falling. The air filled with falling bodies. I
    remember the impact of hitting the trees and the ground.
    When I opened my eyes I knew that I was still alive
    because of the pain of breathing, the pain of feeling my
    body reviving to the breath of life. An old woman had

cushioned my fall and I hated that old woman because she was dead, everybody was dead, and yet I still lived on. I saw Government Māoris coming among the dead. I pulled the old lady and some of the other bodies on top of me so that I would not be seen beneath them. I heard them pull the old lady up and take her scalp. Her blood dripped upon me. Then they were gone.

Scene Four

TIRI *turns to* TILLY.

TIRI: But I lived on. Two others survived. Somebody has to bury the dead. After that was done, we followed after our people and I was reunited with Tamihana and our sons, Ruka and Moanaroa. We made another son — a son for the future. We called him Te Hanene. After the wars the prophet was pardoned. He settled us all at Ohiwa. But one day I saw a rainbow and I thought of those old weavers. I wondered, Who is keeping the fire? I said to Tamihana:

TILLY: I want to go home.

TIRI: To Puketewai?

TILLY: No, to that valley where those old weavers brought me up. It was the only childhood I ever had. It was the only papakāinga I really knew. If you don't want to come, kei te pai. But I have to go. I will take the children with me.

TIRI: E Tiri, do you really think I would let you go and not follow after you? You are like Ruth of the Bible to me. Where you go, I go. Where you make your home, I make my home. Your people are my people, and your god is my god.

TILLY: Then let us take leave of the prophet and journey east.

TIRI: But it wasn't as simple as all that, was it. Don't you remember?

TILLY: It was winter and on our way east Tamihana and the children took sick. Something was wrong with the water. I became sick as well but it's always the woman who has to look after the men and children. All of a sudden I was aware that somebody had come into the room.

> *The theatre flickers with light and shadow. Silver dust sparkles as it falls.*

TILLY: As soon as I saw him, I knew he was Death.

TIRI: He was dark and he came and sat down beside me on the bed. He started to speak to me, but I was trying to cope with staying alive so I said —

TILLY (*laughing, to audience*): You know what she said?

TIRI: Haere atu! Hoki mai koe ki ahau i te toru tekau tau! Oh, go away! I'm too busy right now! Come back in thirty years! (*Scolding* TILLY) It was your idea! You must have *really* frightened him off! (*Calling*) Hey, Death! Can't you count? Where are you, you old deceiver! You're slacking on the job. My bags have been packed for years ... and years ... and ... has the train been delayed?

TILLY: But he did come back, didn't he Tiri? He came back a month later. But not for you, though, eh.

    TIRI *begins to whimper and thresh around.*

TIRI: Why do you do this to me! The memories, the memories ... They are like the spider's web, so strong and tensile that once caught in their strands, nothing, not even Time, can escape them. Men may have big memories of large events. But women's memories are different. They hurt more.

TILLY (*persistent*): Instead of taking you, Death took Tamihana. (*In a mysterious voice*) Where you go, I go?

TIRI (*turning on* TILLY): Yes, you had to do that, didn't you! You had to make out that I was to blame. Well I wasn't, I tell you. A woman never forgets her first man. She never forgets her children. And when a woman buries her man or her children it is as if she has been born to a dark star. These are the occasions by which she marks her history. She would rather that she was burying herself.

    TIRI *chants a waiata tangi for her dead husband.*

    Taka ka taka
    Taka ka taka
    Ka taka te motoi
    E kapo ki te whetū
    E kapo ki te marama
    E kapo ki te ata o taku raukura ka riro –
    Ripiripia! Tihaehaea!
    E a turakina!
    Paranikia te upoko!

Te ngangara kai-tangata, e!
Auē! Auē! Taukiri e!

TILLY *relents and goes to comfort* TIRI *who pushes her away.*

TIRI: After Tamihana died I went to a matakite because I thought she might know the reason why I continued to live while everybody around me died.

TILLY: Oh, young one, you have a lifeline that stretches on forever.

TIRI: But Death has already come for me once —

TILLY: No, you will live on and on.

TIRI: It was she who gave me the name that many people know me by.

TILLY: Ko tō ingoa — Te Wahine Haere Roa.

TIRI: Woman Far Walking.

Scene Five

A loud knocking sound comes over the sound system.

JESSICA (*V/O*): Nani? Are you there? I'm sorry, Nani, I tried to stop them but I can't.

FRED (*V/O*): Jessica? Look, don't try to spoil your nani's birthday. E Kui, are you ready? The television people want to interview you now.

> TIRI *and* TILLY *put their hands to their ears.*

TILLY: God, you look a mess. Couldn't you at least have done your hair before appearing on international television? What an embarrassment you are.

> TILLY *helps* TIRI *out of her coat. She picks up a hand brush and, standing behind the old lady, begins to brush her hair.*

TIRI: Be careful! Kei maro! Don't pull my hair out!

> TILLY *nods. She gets some lipstick and puts some on* TIRI's *lips.*

TIRI: No, don't make me look like a pūkeko.

> TILLY *stands back and looks at her handiwork.*

TILLY: What do you think?

TIRI (*sarcastically*): You forgot the false eyelashes. I don't want to go out there. The world is always waiting. Always asking questions, questions, questions. When I want to forget, I am always forced to remember. I just want to go home. All I ever wanted to do was to go home.

> *On the soundtrack, a rhapsodic flute plays 'Rimurimu'.*

TILLY: After Tamihana died, the children and I carried on eastward. When I saw the valley, I don't know where the feeling came from, but I felt such joy. I ran through the meadow and dived into the stream — and it was like a baptism.

TIRI: Come on, kids! Let's go and find that old whare I used to live in.

TILLY: But, when we got there the whare was no longer standing nor the kāuta. A marae had sprung up overlooking the sea and I went over there. I saw a man storing kūmara in a food house.

TIRI: E koro, what's happened to the old weavers and their brother?

TILLY: Oh, that's such a very sad story. You know, they used to have a young girl who looked after them, but she ran away. Soon after she left, one of the old ladies died. The old man was next. Then the second kuia went. When they were found they were all hugging each other, dead, as if they were trying to keep warm.

   TIRI *begins to weep.*

TIRI (*to* TILLY): You burden me with memories. You are like a pair of pincers squeezing my heart, shredding it. Yet I still live and that heart still pumps my blood, as red as a river. How was I to know?

TILLY: You should have remembered they were not allowed to touch food. Despite what you did to them they left word about who was to inherit the valley —

TIRI: What did they say?

TILLY: The valley, the land, the marae — it's all yours.

TIRI (*with a cry*): I should have stayed —

TILLY (*relenting*): You cannot blame yourself for being a twelve-year-old girl. How were you to know that they would get so feeble that they wouldn't be able to blow on the embers and make a fire to keep them warm?

TIRI *calms down.* TILLY *looks out at the audience.*

But she (*Indicating* TIRI) learnt from that lesson.

TIRI (*to audience*): Oh how I learnt my lesson — I made a vow to those old people. I stooped to the ground and I picked up that sweet soil in my hands and held it to the sky and made my karanga to all the rainbows in the world and the people of the valley to come to me —

> *Back to back, and circling,* TILLY *and* TIRI *begin to call, together and variously, over and over, making the theatre resound with their calls and passion.*

TIRI/TILLY (*in karanga*): Haramai koutou ngā kahukura o te ao, haramai, haramai —

> *Rainbows appear, arching from the stage into the auditorium of the theatre.*

TIRI: And when the rainbows were all in attendance, all gathered there, I made my pact to them —

For as long as I breathe, and as long as I live, this valley and this land is ours and I will fight to keep it forever and ever —

> *Birds begin to sing in a dawn chorus which rises in a crescendo. The sea washes gently on a beach. There is a sense of life renewing itself.*

Act Three

Scene One

TIRI *is sitting, eyes closed, in her wheelchair.* TILLY *is standing behind her. Both have had a costume change, are groomed and look extremely striking. They are wearing long black dresses. They have greenstone earrings and greenstone neck pieces.*

On the soundtrack, waves hiss over the sand and seagulls squeal overhead. The lighting suggests a red sunset, with TIRI *lifting her face to the last rays of the sun.*

JESSICA'*s voice calls to* TIRI.

JESSICA (*V/O*): Nani, are you there?

TIRI (*on stage, murmuring*): I'm here, Jessica.

JESSICA (*V/O*): Will you teach me 'Ka Panapana' Nani?

TIRI: Yes, moko, of course. Hope! Ringawhiuia! Ka panapana!

JESSICA (*V/O*): I a ha ha! Ka rekareka tonu taku ngākau ki ngā mana ririki pōhatu whakapiri —

TIRI: Yes, Jessica. That's right. Sing out loud. The whole world must hear you, moko, everyone in the world —

> JESSICA's *voice fades away as* TIRI *drifts back into her dreams. She begins to make flicking motions as if she was fishing for eels. She shivers in her sleep.*

TILLY (*to audience*): You think she's asleep, don't you! You think that just because she's an old, old lady, she's nodded off. But if she sleeps she dreams — and her dreams are so disturbed. Of blood-red skies and people falling from a cliff. Of seas swirling with kelp and, within the seaweed, the bodies of her babies. The dead pile up at the door of her life. They keep pushing and pushing against the door of her dreams. The only way to keep them out is not to sleep, not to dream. Not to live.

TIRI (*murmuring, recalling the* REPORTER's *question in Act One*): You ask me how I feel, Pākehā? Ancient, that's what. Ugly, that's what. Left behind, that's what. Beached here. Stranded on a beach where the gulls circle, screaming overhead — Die! Die! Die! — and the crabs clack their claws, clack clack clack, waiting for a feast that never comes.

TILLY: The tide, always the tide. But when it ebbs, it does not pull us out with it. We are stranded here. Everyone else has been taken away. Let us go out at the next full moon, at the next tide's ebbing. And you — seagulls — jostling wing-tip to wing-tip, when our time comes, strip us swift, strip us clean to the bone, crowd us, clothe us with your wings, be beak-cruel. Cut, slash, dig, tear, rip, shred. Leave us as bones drying on a beach.

TIRI (*continuing to murmur*): The tide comes in and goes out. Comes in and goes out. I sit on a black rock overlooking the sea and the crabs go clack clack clack, scuttling closer, closer. They know I'm still here – they like to remind me that they have not forgotten we have a date to dine. If I am very still they come right up to the hem of my skirt. They nip at my skin, tasting the flesh that will soon be theirs. (TIRI *opens her eyes. She looks at a member of the audience.*) Did you know that the old time Māori didn't believe in heaven or hell? You worked out your utu, your payment for all you had done in your life, here. Now is your heaven and now is your hell. I have been so cheated of death – (TIRI *turns her attention to her own body. She begins to hit at herself.*) Die, damn you, why don't you die? (TIRI *senses someone behind her. It's* TILLY, *but* TIRI *thinks it's someone else. Without looking*) Is that you, Mum? Have you come to get me? Is it time to go home now?

TILLY: No. It's me.

TIRI (*staring ahead, angry*): It's always you. Why are you always here? What do you want?

TILLY (*stretching her arms out in a pleading fashion*): You know what I want. (*Enigmatically*) What happened was not my fault. I tried not to let it happen. I want you to –

TIRI: Forgive you?

TILLY: Yes.

TIRI: Well, I can't give that to you. I won't give it to you.

TILLY (*smouldering*): So we have to go on to the bitter end?

TIRI: Till Death do us part, girl.

Scene Two

TIRI *stamps her walking sticks on the floor. Front lighting over* TIRI *and* TILLY *suggests the flickering of hundreds of birthday candles.*

CHORUS (*V/O*): Happy birthday to you! Happy birthday to you!
    Happy birthday dear Tiri! Happy birthday to you!

ANGELA (*V/O, giggling*): Here's your cake, Mum dear. I baked it all myself!

FRED (*V/O*): Okay, Kui, blow out your candles.

JESSICA (*V/O*): You shouldn't do this, Daddy.

> *On stage,* TIRI *starts to blow. The lighting dies and then re-lights.* TIRI *blows again. The lighting dies again and re-lights again. On the soundtrack somebody starts to laugh. Others join in. The laughter suddenly cuts off. But on stage, in a panic,* TIRI *continues to blow and blow.* TILLY *calms her down.*

TIRI: Memories are like those candles. You can blow and blow all you like, but they keep coming back ... Those old weavers, they made me a cloak that was so soft that when they put it around my shoulders I felt like a queen. Was it my fault they died? My loved companions, back to back with me against the Pākehā at our cliff-top fortress, Ngatapa. Was I also at fault that they died and I lived? My dear mother ... I was always waiting for her to come to get me. Looking down the road. Even when I was her age, a grown woman, I kept my watch. Instead, it was Life that kept coming down that road. So much life, year after year like one battalion after another going to war! To war! To war!

> TILLY *arches an eyebrow at* TIRI. *She picks up a banjo, tunes it and begins to strum.*

TIRI: You never let me get away with anything, do you?

TILLY: Nope.

TIRI: I got married again. This was in 1882. I was forty-two. Tamihana had been for love. Tainui, he was for laughter.

TILLY: One day he turned up in the valley, plucking on that banjo of his. She was planting maize.

TIRI: Well, don't just stand there! Are you too lazy to hop over the fence. Here, take this shovel and help me!

TILLY: Hey, missus, I am helping! You do the working and I'll do the playing to help you get into the rhythm!

> TILLY *sings 'Oh Susannah' and, as she does so, she makes eyes at* TIRI.

TILLY: Haere mai au i Alabammy
taku banjo on my knee!

> TILLY *pauses to see what effect she is having on* TIRI.

Haere mai au to this valley
ki te kite i a you!
(What's your name, honey?)

TIRI: That's no business of yours!

TILLY: Oh Huhana, kaua e tangi cry just for me
     Haere mai au to this valley
     ki te kite koe for to see!

> TILLY *reprises the song, which is taken up by a small orchestral trio as she does a hoedown. She dances the square dance around* TIRI.

TIRI/TILLY (*harmonising*): Oh Huhana, kaua e tangi cry just
     for me
     Haere mai au to this valley
     Ki te kite koe for to see!

> TIRI *and* TILLY *burst out laughing.*

TIRI: Tainui was hopeless, but was he fun? Was he what! Always singing and making me laugh and tickling my funny bone. I needed to laugh. He ambushed me with his humour.

TILLY: His body more like it! (*As* TAINUI) What you grieving for, girl! What the long face for! (*Begins to sing and snap her fingers*) You got to get back into life, forget all your personal strife and live, live, live! You got to get back into love, you ain't been no turtle dove (I can tell you's a real woman who needs a laughing man) and love, love, love!

TIRI: God he was a real runt.

TILLY: Ugly as.

TIRI: Came up only to our shoulders.

TILLY: As far as that? The only problem was —

TIRI: He could sure sneak up on you when you weren't looking. And two kids later —

TILLY: Oh Huhana, kaua e tangi cry just for me!
Haere mai au i Alabammy —

> TILLY *stops in mid-song.* TIRI *has fallen silent. She begins to stalk* TIRI *around the set.*

TIRI: You think you can fox me with good memories, ne? Well you can't.

TILLY: Leave me alone, Kui. You just leave me alone —

TIRI: You talk about the two children. What about the third one, eh? The pale child. Pirimia. You shouldn't have had it. You should have done something to it.

> *A half moon rises in the sky. There is a replay on the soundtrack of the birth scene from Act One. However, instead of* TIRI *chanting an oriori she chants a pātere, a song of scorn and anger.*

TILLY: Auē te mamae!

> TIRI's *voice overrides* TILLY's.

TIRI: Auē te hē! Auē te hē!

> TIRI *has a knife in her hands. She goes to* TILLY *with the knife.*

TIRI: Here. Take it.

TILLY: The smell of a newborn child —

TIRI: Look at it. Captain Cook looked like this. A pale child.
A goblin's child with eyes at the back of its head —

TILLY: The feel of one's own flesh against your skin —

TIRI: Can you not see and smell the child?

> TIRI *pushes the knife into* TILLY's *hands. She advances on* TILLY, *her voice and attitude determined.*

TIRI: Do it before it's too late. Kill it. Kill it!

> *On the soundtrack, there is the sound of a child's wail.* TILLY *sways. She drops the knife. It clatters on the floor.* TILLY *crumples in a heap, sobbing.*

TIRI: You were weak. You should have killed it —

> TIRI *spins her wheelchair away in a rage. She mimes flicking a line, and then throwing the line away. She mimes blowing out candles again and again. She is spiralling, turning her wheelchair around and around in an attempt to escape.*

TIRI (*helplessly*): They keep on coming back, the memories,
coming back. (*With a sudden change of mood*) Unlike Death,
of course, he didn't come back. (*Calling out*) I told you to
return in thirty years! Too busy elsewhere? Asleep on the
job?

> TILLY *recovers from the trauma of her last scene.*

TILLY: Oh, don't pretend to be offended. When he didn't
come when he was supposed to you went dancing around
the house as if you'd cheated him at cards and won.

TIRI: Maybe, but I didn't expect to keep on living for so long after that! On and on and on. Especially by 1918 I was ready to die but I didn't. Yet, everybody else — (*Hides her face*) Oh, I don't want to tell them.

Scene Three

TIRI *stares upward, into the auditorium. All of a sudden, gunfire crackles. The explosions of Allied and enemy bombardment sound on the soundtrack. The lighting simulates the Great War of 1914-18, biplanes overhead, bombs exploding and shadows advancing across No Man's Land.*

SOLDIER (*V/O*): Are you ready, men? Bayonets at the ready! At the count of three I want you over the side! One, two, three — Charge!

TIRI: 1914. Another war. The Great War. Always war.

> TIRI *and* TILLY *stare into the darkness as if witnessing the war. A bugle sounding the attack. Allied and enemy soldiers engaging in hand-to-hand combat.*

TIRI: Turuki, turuki, paneke paneke —

TILLY: Look at them all. Rifles at the ready. Charging through the barbed wire. Listen to the chatter of the machine-guns. The soldiers soon too die, staggering through the mud and corpses of those already dead —

TIRI: Tumatauenga, the god of war, reaps a rich harvest.

TILLY: Look, Kui. Gas –

> *Smoke curls across the floor of the stage.* TIRI *and* TILLY
> *put white handkerchiefs to their mouths and nose as if to*
> *protect themselves from the gas. The enemy bombard-*
> *ment, the cries of the dying and other sounds fade away.*

TILLY: We were seventy-eight in 1918 when the Great War
ended.

TIRI: Were we that old already?

TILLY: We had grown really old. So had Tainui. (*Mysteriously*)
We had found – peace – with each other. Our children
had grown up. The only shadow on our happiness was
that Moanaroa and Pirimia had enlisted to fight in the
First World War. We didn't want them to go.

TIRI: Why should I let you go to fight with the Pākehā?

TILLY: Everybody's going, Māmā.

TIRI: I've been fighting him all my life! I was Te Kooti's left
hand of God against him. And you tell me you want to go
and fight for him?

TILLY: We'll be fighting against the Germans, Māmā.

TIRI: Good. Let the Pākehā fight the Pākehā. Goblin against
goblin. Maybe they'll kill each other. You boys are staying
home.

> *A silence.* TILLY *approaches* TIRI.

TILLY: But you know what boys are like. They want to be

warriors. They want to have a glorious battle. It doesn't matter what the war —

TIRI: Yes it *does*. And look what happened. Moanaroa died there in Europe, killed at the Somme. The one who should have died, Pirimia, he came home.

> *On the soundtrack we hear a train coming into a railway station. People are cheering and a military band playing a waltz – the First World War Māori tune 'E Pari Rā'.*

TILLY: Can you see him? Can you see Pirimia?

TIRI: Oh no, is that the mayor getting up to speak? We'll be here all day —

TILLY (*as* MAYOR): Not all of our boys have come back. Over 15,000 lie in foreign fields. In France, at Flanders. In Turkey, at Gallipoli. Along the Western Front. They gave up their lives so that we might live. Some of our own boys, our farmer boys, were among them. The Richardson lads. The Connor boys. The McTavish sons. My own boy James. We shall not forget them. But we the living must go on. And this is not only a time for sadness but also joy that most of our lads have made it back home. Three cheers for our boys —

> *The soundtrack echoes with cheers of 'Hurrah!'*

TIRI (*remembering*): Of course the mayor forgot to mention *our* Māori boys. Nor did he talk about the other *thing*, the *mate*, that had come back on the train as well.

TILLY (*nodding*): It was only later, two days later, when some of the boys began to turn black that we realised —

TIRI: I had a bad dream, an omen. Pirimia, the pale son, was in my dream. I had to sprinkle myself with water and pray very hard. Tainui asked me, 'He aha te mate?' I couldn't tell him. It was Pirimia who brought the flu to us. The night he arrived home we had a huge welcome and he kissed everybody. It was the kiss of death. Our village, at that time, must have been about ninety-six men, women and children.

> TILLY *takes on the role of Pirimia and begins to cough. Both she and* TIRI *put white handkerchiefs to their faces. Realisation comes to* TILLY'S *face that she has the flu. She pushes* TIRI *away.*

TIRI: What's wrong with you?

TILLY: Oh my god, you must all keep away from me. All of you. Keep away.

TIRI: There was a gurgling sound. His body gave a series of violent contractions. Then a thick black fluid spouted out of his mouth. We didn't know what he was talking about. By the time we realised, it was too late.

> TILLY *switches a radio on. Through the static comes a* NEWSREADER'S *voice.* TIRI'S *dialogue goes over the news report. Smoke begins to curl again over the stage.*

NEWSREADER (*V/O*): And now news about the Spanish influenza which is sweeping the Dominion. Over 100 Auckland citizens have died from the flu, which has now reached epidemic proportions. In the capital and in Christchurch, schools and theatres have closed down. There is a ban on tangis. Citizens are urged to limit all congress with the Māori population ...

TIRI: My dream, my premonition, was coming true. By the third day, at least half of the village was down with the sickness. Somehow, I was spared. Why me? I don't know. I guess that there have to be some among the living who have to be spared to bury the dead —

> *The radio crackles with static and begins a second broadcast. Meanwhile,* TILLY *screams at the sight of the curling smoke, like mist, and is trying to escape from it.*

NEWSREADER (*V/O*): The death toll from the Spanish influenza continues to rise, and reports from the rest of the world have led experts to estimate that over 15 million have died so far. New Zealand has not escaped the ravages of the epidemic. People are asked to remain in their homes —

TIRI (*to audience*): The war was over but we were still at war —

> TIRI *chants 'Turuki turuki, paneke paneke' over the continuation of the* NEWSREADER's *reportage. The soundtrack reprises the baying horns heard earlier during the Matawhero Retaliation in Act Two. The lighting takes on a sickly green effect.*

NEWSREADER (*V/O*): At least six thousand New Zealanders are expected to succumb to the disease. Three thousand have already died. No statistics have come in regarding the Māori population but there is no doubt that their insanitary living conditions and susceptibility to diseases will mean that they will be hard hit. Authorities continue to advise that under no circumstances should —

In a temper, TIRI *turns on the audience. She advances through the smoke.*

TIRI (*addressing the audience*): You, Pākehā, you have always wanted us to die, haven't you, and this was your way how to do it. We tried to take our sick to the hospitals and you put up roadblocks to prevent us. Wherever we went, north, south, east and west, you trapped us and kept us imprisoned. You, Pākehā, you refused us medical supplies. Yes, and you, Pākehā, in the end you said it was us who had caused the flu.

TIRI beckons TILLY *to come to her.* TILLY *is nervous, trying not to let the smoke cling to her. Together,* TIRI *and* TILLY *enact boiling water, miming blowing on the fire, stripping sheets for bandages and so on.*

TILLY: They used to call me the keeper of the fire. All my life I have been the one to blow on the embers and to keep the fire alight.

TIRI (*to* TILLY): We have to isolate the ill from the ones who are not yet ill. The flu is a bacteria which attacks the lungs. The bacteria is passed from one person to another when that person breathes it in. Flu patients will cough, then they will spit phlegm and blood. They suffer high fevers. If we keep their temperatures down, they have a chance. If we don't —

Suddenly TILLY *backs away.*

What's wrong with you, girl!

TILLY: Tainui, look at Tainui. Oh Huhana, kaua e tangi cry just for me —

TIRI (*to audience*): Why did it have to be Tainui? He never did anything to anybody? Why did it have to happen to my laughing man? He started to cough. I held him so tight as I heard his breath rattling around in his chest. All of a sudden he gave a gasp, spouted blood from his throat and turned ... he turned ... *black* —

TILLY: It is the colour of sin —

TIRI: Then *you* should be the one to go black, not him. You are the one who should have received God's punishment. You should be wearing the mark of Cain. You —

> TILLY *reprises the waiata tangi that* TIRI *earlier chanted from Act Two.*

TILLY: Taka ka taka
Taka ka taka
He falls he falls
The greenstone pendant falls
I snatch at the star
I snatch at the moon
I snatch at the shadow
of my lost feather plume,
Ripiripia! Tihaehaea!
Ripiripia! Tihaehaea!
Auē! Taukiri e!

> TILLY *continues to mourn.* TIRI *looks at her, unforgiving. The wind begins to howl on the soundtrack. The wind blows the smoke like sand blowing across sand dunes.*

TIRI: No excuses. No time to say goodbye. One minute there. The next minute gone. (*To* TILLY) Here, put his body on a sled. We have to take his body to the sand dunes. Bury him in the sand. Deep, deep so the dogs won't dig him up. So the Pākehā won't get at him, won't desecrate him. Deep, deep, away from your secret —

> *During the foregoing,* TILLY *is buckling a harness to her shoulders. The harness is attached to a sled.*

TILLY: Yes, that's right. Kick me while I'm down. That's all you know about, isn't it? (*Whistling, as if to a dog*) Come on, kurī, we have to get some water from the stream —

TILLY *exits, pulling the sled.*

TIRI (*to audience*): She stirs up my memories, this is what she gets. If she can't take it, get out of the kitchen. Let her suffer. She's to blame! Not just for Tainui but also for those others who died. From our village and from other villages. I would see them from afar coming across the sandhills to bury *their* dead —

The wind is whistling, the sand blowing. TIRI *mimes looking across the sand dunes. In the distance,* TILLY *is pulling the sled.*

TIRI: Tokohia ngā mate o tō kāinga? How many dead in your village?

TILLY: Tekau! Ten! Rua tekau! Twenty! Toru tekau —

TIRI: As the weeks went by, the toll mounted. Forty. Fifty. Seventy —

TILLY *exits with the sled. The smoke stops blowing.*

TIRI: When I didn't see those people coming across the sandhills any more I knew all of them had gone. Even those who had lived to bury the dead. Over the radio we heard that if you survived seven days of the flu you were likely to survive it. So I said to some of the younger ones, the healthy ones, Haere atu! Haere atu koutou ki roto i te ngahere, noho ai. Go into the bush away from here where the flu can't get you. When it's over, come back. There were five of them. Two were just kids, six years old. They didn't want to go. The others were teenagers, two young girls and one boy.

The lights simulate a lightning strike. TILLY *returns as if unwrapping herself from dreams.*

NEWSREADER (*V/O*): The Spanish influenza rages on throughout the world and the Commonwealth. Experts now predict that an estimated 21 million will die. Reports from Western Samoa suggest that half of the male population are already affected.

   Grave fears, however, are held for the native population. The native ministers, Maui Pomare, Apirana Ngata and Peter Buck have all reported high death rates, particularly in the Taranaki and the Waikato. At last report ...

   TIRI *stamps her walking sticks on the floor. The lightning clears.*

TIRI: At last report? At last report? I have seen too much death. All my loved ones, gone. And I am still here, alone, the last of my kind, and desolate on the shore.

TILLY: But you were not alone. There were others who survived. Our son, Pirimia —

TIRI (*suddenly*): Don't you dare to call him our son. He was *your* son.

TILLY: ... was one. The five who ran into the bush, they survived. Two other girls —

TIRI: Nine out of ninety-six?

TILLY: Some people say we were lucky —

TIRI: Lucky? There is nothing lucky about living on when everybody else is gone. The tide comes in and goes out. Comes in and goes out.

TILLY: A few weeks later, the first Pākehā came into our area to see how we were.

> TIRI *mimes digging graves with a shovel.*

TILLY: The Pākehā looked like they were spacemen from the moon. We were still burying our dead in the sand. (*To* TIRI) Did you ever see such eyes, Tiri, blue like a devil's? This toeless imprint?

> TILLY *backs away.* TIRI *moves forward. On the sound-track comes the sounds associated with the coming of history that Pākehā settlement brought with it.*

VOICES (*V/O*): Huihuingia mai rā ō tātou mate! Huihuingia! Au! Au! Au! Au!

TIRI: I suppose you're the cavalry.

TILLY: Do you need help?

TIRI: Te mātauranga a te Pākehā he mea whakatō mō wai rā? Mō Hātana! Mō Hātana! You brought your plague upon us. This is my valley. We bury our own. Now get out. (TIRI *throws the shovel to one side. She stands in her wheelchair and takes a few steps forward towards the audience, as if to the edge of a grave.*) Why me, you fullas? Why leave me behind? Tainui? All of you? You think I'm the strong one, is that it? Must I always be the keeper of the fire? Is this my punishment for letting it go out when those old weavers died? You think it's easy for me to bury all of you? Useless pakas! Can't do a thing for yourselves! Always leaving me to clean up after you! Leaving me to look after your kids! Why me? (*Signing to* TILLY) Burn the village down. We must rid the houses of the plague –

> *All of a sudden there is a boom and the lighting simulates flickering flames dancing higher and higher.* TIRI *is caught up in a torrent of emotion.* TILLY *is running around the stage, trying to get away.*

TILLY: I'm not to blame. Tiri, don't. Please stop. Please.

TIRI (*to her dead*): I want you all to come back. Come back, do you hear? Me hoki mai koutou. Me hoki ... mai ... koutou.

> TIRI*'s grief ends. She motions* TILLY *to join her.*

TIRI: We can't stay here. There's not enough of us.

TILLY: Āe, let's go north. We have kin we can stay with.

TIRI (*as if she is speaking to the survivors*): So only nine of us, eh? Ah well, where there is one there is a thousand. Where there are nine, there can be ninety or nine hundred or nine thousand! All of you have the blood of your whānau in your veins. You start making babies, you hear me! You bring the bloodlines back. You make sure these people didn't die for nothing. You hear me? And then you come back here and rebuild the valley. Where there's one there's a thousand. You hear me? A thousand —

The flames dance and burn. The soundtrack crackles with the sound of the flames.

Act Four

Scene One

The flames from Act Three form a bridge to Act Four. TIRI *and* TILLY *return to the 'doorway' position on the set.* TILLY *helps* TIRI *to change into her white dressing gown.* TILLY *pulls on jeans. On the soundtrack we hear a voice in French.*

VOICE *(V/O)*: En garde! Alerte! Dix, neuf, huit, septe, six, cinq, quatre, trois, deux, un —

> *The countdown heightens the tension on stage.*

TILLY: We must hurry —

TIRI: Will Jessica be all right?

TILLY: Kia tere! Kia tere!

> *But* TIRI *and* TILLY *are too late. As they continue to change clothes there is a huge roar followed by all those sounds associated with a nuclear blast. The lighting simulates the blast — a white sheet of light which fills the entire auditorium.*

TIRI (*shouting*): Jessica —

> *The impact goes over* TIRI *and* TILLY *and they put their arms up to their eyes to protect themselves from the sheer intensity of the light.*

RADIO ANNOUNCER (*V/O*): This morning at 0700 hours the French Government completed its third round of nuclear tests on Moruroa Atoll. The New Zealand Government has joined all Pacific nations in protesting to the French at the continuation of the tests —

> *During the foregoing* TIRI *and* TILLY *are chanting their way to the front of the stage in a similar fashion to their entrance to Act Two.*

TIRI: When my grandmother saw Captain Cook come sailing into Tolaga she said he looked like a goblin. Wherever he goes he murders people. The Americas. The Africas. Polynesia. He murders even his own. What kind of goblin does that? Now he murders the land and the sea. We must not let him. To war! To war!

TILLY (*gently*): From your wheelchair, Left Hand of God? It's not just your battle now. And you are so old. So old.

> TIRI'*s anger subsides. She begins to sigh to herself.*

TIRI: After we left the valley, how long did we stay with our relations?

TILLY: Many years. We stayed with Pirimia in Auckland. Remember? In 1940 we were one hundred years old.

TIRI (*smiling*): One hundred. *Scary*.

TILLY: We had become the last of our generation. Of our children, there was only Pirimia – and he died just after World War Two.

TIRI: Yes, I remember Pirimia dying. I tried to cry for him but I couldn't –

TILLY: Our granddaughter, Arihia, took us in.

TIRI: I remember. When we told her we might want to go back to the valley she put her foot down.

TILLY: Who's going to look after you in a valley that you can't even get to by road! No, you're staying here and that's that.

TIRI: Oh, Arihia was a lovely girl but her husband – no good. And what happened after that? The memories march over me like soldiers.

TILLY: We stayed with Arihia until 1957. When *she* died her eldest son, Rawiri, he took us in. It was him and his wife, Joanna, who brought us to Wellington. The city of gold. There were more opportunities. More jobs. More money.

TIRI: Ah yes. (*Contemptuously, rubbing her fingers*) Money. Were there babies? *Were* there!

TILLY: Our whānau were fruitful. From the nine did indeed come ninety – and there are many more now. The winds have scattered them to other cities. Even overseas to Sydney. You have some mokopuna living in Los Angeles now.

TIRI (*stamping her walking sticks*): Did any go back to the valley? *Did* they!

TILLY: Yes. They have a pub, a place where you can rent videos and a Lotto shop up there now.

> TIRI *nods with relief and then glares at* TILLY. *She pokes* TILLY *with a walking stick.*

TIRI: Somewhere along the line somebody found out about my age and told King George the Sixth! Was it you?

TILLY: Me? Why would I want to be part of this circus! Every Waitangi Day, journalists with their stupid questions. 'To what do you attribute your longevity, Mrs Mahana?'

TIRI: Regular bowel movements.

TILLY: 'And why do you think you've lived so long?'

TIRI: I have sex every day.

TILLY: 'And what words of wisdom would you like to leave for the younger generation?'

TIRI: Remember that when Ginger Rogers danced with Fred Astaire she did everything he did but she did it backwards *and* in high heels.

> TIRI *and* TILLY *burst into joint laughter. After a moment,* TIRI *begins to make the flicking motion. For the rest of the act she flicks between reality and dream, past and present, laughter and tears. She is, after all, at the extremes of age and the burden of all her memories pushes her often into a state similar to dementia.*

TIRI (*sighing*): Oh, I loved that Ginger when she danced on the screen. (*Pauses, looking at* TILLY) As for you, it must have been you who blabbed. Before King George died he told his daughter, Elizabeth, and I'm still on somebody's list to get a royal telegram. Has it arrived yet?

TILLY: No. But the news media, television and everybody, is still out there, waiting for it. Your command performance, darling.

TIRI: Can't you tell them all to go away and leave me alone? No matter where I am, no matter where I go, somebody is always watching me. Always. They pursue me like gulls crowding the sky — like black crabs clack clack clacking on the rocks where the tide surges. And, no matter where I look, all that life, that history, keeps coming at me, coming down the road.

TILLY: You're forgetting your mokopuna, Mere —

> TILLY *begins to put on a motorbike jacket and dark shades.*

TIRI: Mere? Rawiri's daughter? How can you ask if I have forgotten her? I will never forget Mere! If it hadn't been for her I would have spent most of my days watching television in my room. Watching the world go past. The 60s. The 70s. Before I knew it, it was the 1980s and my next war was just waiting around the corner.

Scene Two

The soundtrack begins to clatter with the sound of helicopters circling in the auditorium.

RADIO ANNOUNCER (*V/O*): Good morning, Vietnam!

> *The soundtrack then begins a short montage of excerpts from popular songs of the 50s, 60s and 70s.*

SOUNDTRACK: Good, good, good, good vibrations! Que sera sera, whatever will be, will be! Come on baby, light my fire! Do you know the way to San Jose? It's been a hard day's night and I've been working like a dog! Up up and away, in my beautiful, my beautiful balloon —

> *The lights change to disco.* TILLY *strikes a pose.*

TIRI (*with a gasp of love*): Is that you, Mere? Have you come to my birthday too?

TILLY *makes an entrance miming and dancing to Nancy Sinatra's 'These Boots are Made for Walking'. She circles and bops around the set and struts her stuff around* TIRI.

TILLY: Okay, boots! Start walkin' —

> TILLY *gives* TIRI *a high five.*

Kia ora, Nan! Don't you get sick and tired of sitting in the dark looking at bad television? Come on! Come with me!

TIRI: On your motorbike? Hoi! You don't think I'm getting on the back of that!

TILLY: Oh, live dangerously, Nan! Here, let me help you tuck your dress in your pants, and off we go!

> TILLY *pretends* TIRI's *wheelchair is a motorbike.* TILLY *pushes* TIRI *all over the set, miming the motion of speeding along the highway and leaning into the curves. On the soundtrack, the sound of a motorbike revving up and down.*

TIRI: Where we going today?

TILLY: To Raglan, to help those Waikato people to get their land back. (*To audience*) Not one more acre of Māori land! Honour the Treaty!

TIRI: And after Raglan?

TILLY: I thought you might like to go on a little walk —

TIRI: Ha! *Little* walk she says. All the way from Te Hapua across the Auckland Harbour Bridge to Wellington!

TILLY (*to audience*): The Treaty is a fraud! Māori sovereignty! (*Imitating the noise of a motorbike*) Kia ora, Nani! We're having a *little* meeting at university. Do you want to come along?

TIRI: As long as I drive!

TILLY: Well, um —

TIRI: Don't you want to live dangerously?

> TILLY *laughs and nods.*

TILLY: Watch out! Look out for that truck! Slow down, Nani! Do you want to get us killed?

TIRI: Hmm. What a good idea —

TILLY (*singing*): Up up and away, in my beautiful my beautiful balloon! Akona te reo Māori!

> *The soundtrack fills with screeching brakes and horns blaring.* TILLY *puts her hands over her eyes.*

TILLY: Are we there?

TIRI: Yup! Faster than a speeding bullet! Quicker than liquid lightning! It's a bird!

TILLY: It's a plane!

TIRI: It's —

TILLY: Super Nan!

TIRI (*to audience*): I guess you could say that Mere was the last big love of my life. Her dad, Rawiri, used to scold her. They used to try to stop me from going with her. Sometimes they'd try to send her away.

TILLY: Mere, your kuia is 140 years old! She's much too old to be out on the streets with you, all day and all night — and last week she got a ticket for dangerous driving!

TIRI: But you never listened to them, eh Mere. You would come around to the back window.

TILLY (*whistling softly*): Hey! Super Nan! Let's go while they're not looking!

TIRI (*to audience*): Did I forget to tell you that Arihia's house was an upstairs and downstairs and I was in an upstairs bedroom? (*Calling*) How am I going to get down there from up here!

TILLY: Easy! See that drainpipe?

TIRI: No way. You go and find a ladder.

> TIRI *and* TILLY *mime helping each other down a ladder. They put on their helmets.*

TIRI: So where are we going today? E haere ana tāua ki hea?

TILLY: To the airport —

TIRI: What for?

TILLY: It's 1981, Nan, and the Springbok rugby team is arriving. They're all White, Nan. Their country legislates against the Black man. We have to stop the Tour.

> *On the soundtrack we hear the shrieking sound as a jet plane lands. Voices begin to yell.*

VOICES (*V/O*): Stop the Tour! Muldoon out! Stop the Tour!

TILLY (*looking across at* TIRI): Oh, we had fun, didn't we Nan? During those Tour protests! Running out onto the field at Hamilton —

TIRI: We could still run —

TILLY: The Test in Auckland —

TIRI (*to audience*): Some of our mongrel relations were going into the game and there were we outside haranguing them. And the police were in front of us, but Mere was so staunch.

TILLY: Hey, you fullas! Remember Steve Biko! Hey, Mister Māori Policeman, you're on the wrong side! And don't you give me the glad eye, Pākehā, or I'll set my grandmother onto you — and she bites!

TIRI: I was so proud of you, Mere. You made me remember all my battles. Some of your Pākehā colleagues said to you —

TILLY: Mere, don't you think your great-great-grandmother is a bit too old for this?

TIRI: But we loved a good fight, eh. I can still remember what you replied. You looked across at me and you beamed this strong, golden smile —

TILLY: E Kui, isn't it a nice day to go for a walk in the sun?

TIRI: Turuki turuki, paneke paneke! Turuki turuki, paneke paneke!

> *The soundtrack explodes into chanting. TIRI and TILLY approach the front of the stage. The lighting allows TIRI and TILLY to cast shadows which convey other people in the background.*

TIRI/ TILLY/SOUNDTRACK: Amandla! Amandla ngawhetu!

> *The action is continuous as TIRI and TILLY execute choreographed movements to the chant. The movements are spectacular and like a dance, Māori movements based on the wero.*
> *Over the top of the chanting comes the voice of Kiri Te Kanawa singing 'Let The Bright Seraphim' at Prince Charles and Lady Diana's wedding.*

KIRI TE KANAWA (*V/O*): Let the bright seraphim ...

> *Finally the music is taken up another notch by the addition of fragments from the massacre at Ngatapa and the 1918 flu epidemic. By this point the music is at overload.*

POLICE SQUAD (*V/O*): Red squad at the ready! This is your last warning. Retreat and disperse peacefully. No? Batons at the ready! Hold your ranks. Advance –

TIRI/TILLY (*over everything*): Kia kaha! Kia manawanui! E tū! Nekeneke! Au! Au! Au! Au!

> *The sequence is still continuous as the lighting suggests the police preparing to make a baton charge against protesters at Molesworth Street. A kettledrum begins to roll.*

VOICE (*V/O, suggesting the soldiers at Ngatapa*): Shoulder, aim, fire!

> *The batoning begins. People scream. Dame Kiri's voice still rides through the soundtrack.*

TILLY (*to* TIRI): Here, Nan, you better have my helmet –

> *TILLY mimes being batoned. She spins and spins as if trying to ward off batons. She is hit and sinks to the ground. Immediately, TIRI is cradling her. The lighting and violence diminishes. The last sound to be heard is Dame Kiri's voice coming to the triumphant conclusion of the aria. Silence.*

TIRI: When I opened my eyes I knew I was still alive. I knew because of the pain of breathing, the pain of feeling my body reviving to the breath of life. I saw that an old woman had cushioned my fall. I hated that old woman because I knew she was dead, that everybody was dead, that my children were dead, shot between the eyes and, yet, I still lived on. Then I saw that Government Māori were coming among the dead scalping them for money, and I pulled the old lady on top of me, and the blood dripped, the blood dripped —

> TIRI *stands up. She looks down at* TILLY. *Her dream world is in full fragmentation between past and present, reality and unreality.*

E tū, kurī, get up! Get up! (*Sways and recovers*) Sometimes the memories flow like a river. The currents cross and re-cross, and when the passions are in full flood they join, swollen, together. You live this long, these things happen. Reality and unreality. Yesterday and today. Madness and sanity. One minute there. Next minute gone.

> TILLY *stands.*

TIRI/TILLY: But *you* still live on and all that life, all that history, is like waves of the sea bursting above you, curling you down into the sand. But somehow, you always find yourself bursting above the waves again, raw with the need to breathe in the air. Even if you don't want it, your body is traitorous. It forces you to fight for breath — madness. People only remember the big events of history. But for a woman, history is intimate. It has to do with the birth of children, grandchildren, great-grand-children —

TIRI: Great-great-great-grandchildren —

TILLY: It has to do with whooping cough, the first steps a child takes, the triumphs and failures of their lives. It has to do with supporting them, holding them when they are dying —

TIRI (*indicating* TILLY): My lovely Mere. She was never the same after that. Something broke inside her head. She sometimes had these dizzy spells, these big headaches. And one day, as she was speeding on her motorbike she was in an accident. I went to see her in hospital.

TILLY: Faster than a speeding bullet — Super Nan... Akona te reo Māori. Not one more acre of Māori land. Māori land for Māori people. When I die will you take me back to our rainbow valley and will you bury me in the sand with my ancestors?

TIRI: Yes, I promise you —

TILLY: I better put on my boots, Nan. (*Sings*) These boots were made for walkin'... One of these days these boots ...

TIRI (*to audience*): I loved that girl. When she died like that I didn't want to go on by myself. Blowing on the fire every morning. Covering the fire every night. I saw people going across the sand dunes and I called out to them, How many left in your village? How many? How *many* —

> TIRI *breaks down. She clasps her abdomen, remembering the babies that have come from her womb.* TIRI *reprises* 'Rimurimu'.

TIRI/TILLY: Rimurimu, tere tere, ki te moana!
Tere ana ki te ripo i waho e!

Tirohia atu ki waho rā, marino ana e!
Kei roto i ahau, marangai ana e —
Kei te tio te huka, i runga o ngā hiwi!
Kei te moe koromeke te wairua e!
Rite tonu tō hanga ki te tīrairaka e!
Waihoki tō hanga, te wairangi e ...

At the end of the waiata TIRI *looks at the audience.*

TIRI: Is survival all that a woman ever knows? That we have to keep going, that it all has to do with keeping on going? Keeping on going on? Always onward, and onward? Is this the role of women?

Scene Three

Flickering lights and shadow. The sound of a royal fanfare. TIRI *starts, gathers in her energy for the final part of the play.* TILLY *also gathers her energy.* TIRI *stamps her walking sticks on the floor.*

TILLY: Our birthdays kept on happening. We were passed —

TIRI: Like a parcel —

TILLY: To Fred and his wife Angela.

TIRI: The current jailers —

TILLY: In 1990 we celebrated our 150th birthday. Jessica told us the Queen was coming to Waitangi.

TIRI (*calling out*): Fred? Fred!

FRED (*V/O*): What's wrong, Kui?

TIRI: Put me in your car and take me up to Waitangi. I want to celebrate my birthday up there this year.

TILLY: They were delighted. They thought this was their chance to meet the Queen. Little did they know that we had something else on our mind. After all were we not the left hand of God?

> *The soundtrack introduces the hubbub of a Waitangi Day gathering.*

ANGELA (*V/O*): Fred, dear, who's that old lady walking out in front of the Queen?

FRED (*V/O*): Oh shit, it's the kuia.

ANGELA (*V/O*): Jessica! Go out there and bring your nani back.

JESSICA (*V/O*): Go, Nan!

> TIRI *faces the audience as if she is on the treaty grounds.*

TIRI (*to the Queen*): You are the Queen of England. You are the white heron. You have flown over every valley of this land, and where your shadow has been thrown, there the land has been taken. I was named after the Treaty which your forefathers signed to guarantee our ownership. You have failed us. You have dishonoured my name. You have broken the Treaty —

TILLY: And after that little exhibition guess who was stripped, like a teenager, of all her privileges!

TIRI: Placed on curfew —

TILLY: Not allowed to see boys —

TIRI: Kept at home and denied access to the telephone —

TILLY: Not allowed to go dancing —

TIRI: The only joy in my life has been Jessica. How she ever came from such boring parents is one of those twists of fate beyond anyone's understanding.

TILLY: But we were lucky, weren't we, Kui, that Jessica was on our side.

TIRI (*nodding*): Yes, she dobbed her parents in.

TILLY: After we had returned from Waitangi she told us:

JESSICA (*V/O*): Nan, are you listening? Nani? I heard Dad talking. He's sold the rights of the ironsand in our valley. He's sold them to the Japanese. They're going to start mining the sand next week. Shipping it to Japan.

> *A moment's silence.* TILLY *has walked a few paces away — and turns, a mocking smile on her face.*

TILLY: Now see how you like being kicked when you're down. Had enough, old lady?

TIRI: One of my own is doing this? One of my own?

TILLY (*mocking*): Calm down, old lady! What do we need the valley for! There's nothing there of use to anybody —

TIRI: Nothing? Nothing? I was given that land in trust by old weavers. People have lived and died on that land. Our bones are buried there. The old weavers. Tamihana.

Tainui. All my children. All their children and children's children. My beloved Mere. Our people are in the sand. They were never safe in their lives from the goblin Pākehā – are they now not safe even in death? All my life I have fought the Pākehā and his Satanic ways! Must he put his mark on every piece of land? And must one of my own connive to help him in this? Never. I made a vow to those old people. My job has always been to keep the fire alight. Ahi kā! Ahi kā –

> *On the soundtrack we hear finally, in focus, the sounds associated with the history that Pākehā settlement has brought with it. The sounds centre on the roar of bull-dozers and huge earth-moving equipment.*
> TIRI *calls into the auditorium.*

TIRI: Jessica, haramai!

TILLY (*V/O*): I'm afraid, Nani.

TIRI: Don't you worry, grandchild. I've faced worse than this.

JESSICA: But what happens if they don't stop?

TIRI: There're no buts. We must make them stop. (TIRI *extends her arms wide in a movement which shows that she is in the path of the tractors. The sound of the tractors rolls from the back of the auditorium towards the stage. As it approaches the stage,* TIRI *takes a few steps forward – she has always confronted her challenges. She makes peruperu movements with her walking stick.*) Get back! Get back –

> *A dramatic silence. From the stage* TILLY *starts to karanga.*

TILLY: Haramai koutou ngā kahukura o te ao, haramai, haramai —

TIRI (*joining in*): Haramai, haramai, haramai —

A rainbow appears. TIRI *turns to* TILLY.

TIRI: When I die, don't bury me in the ground. Burn me up. I don't want to end up in Japan, do you hear? And don't put me in the sea, either. All those fishing trawlers, they might catch me and I'll end up as fish fillet. You hear me? Do you hear? If we don't stop them, burn me up. You'll hear all about it if you don't burn me up —

Scene Four

TIRI *and* TILLY *are spent and exhausted.*

TIRI: Jessica?

JESSICA (*V/O*): Yes, Nani?

TIRI: You remember the women's haka? 'Ka Panapana'?

JESSICA (*V/O*): Yes, Nan.

TIRI: It is your song, moko. For as long as you breathe, sing it out loud. For as long as you live, fight to keep our valley forever and ever. You must be the keeper of the fire —

JESSICA (*V/O*): Yes, Nani. Ake, ake, ake —

TIRI's eyes narrow. She seems to be trying to make up her mind about something. She looks at TILLY. The moment is dangerous. Her voice comes quietly out of nowhere.

TIRI: Now, you. It's time we had it out. We have some unfinished business to settle. (*In a low, purposeful voice*) You wanna fight?

TILLY looks at TIRI and spits on her hands. She picks up two peruperu sticks and throws one to TIRI. TIRI uses the wheelchair as her support. TIRI and TILLY begin a peruperu duel. They test each other out, feinting, trying to find ways through each other's defenses. TILLY is winning when TIRI introduces the memory that has always been hidden.

TIRI (*to* TILLY): You like to make me remember. Here's something you should remember. You've been so hot on my telling the truth, the whole truth and nothing but the truth. Well let's see how you like it.

Flickering shadows and light. In the distance, the horns begin to bray, similar in sound to those used for the Matawhero Retaliation sequence. TILLY begins to whimper and back away from TIRI. She runs everywhere, trying to find a way out. TIRI stalks her.

FIRST MALE VOICE (*V/O*): Is this the place?

SECOND MALE VOICE (*V/O*): Yeah, her husband's out.

THIRD MALE VOICE (*V/O*): So who's first?

FOURTH MALE VOICE (*V/O*): Me —

> TIRI *presses home her attack as the soundtrack graph-*
> *ically conveys the sounds of four men breaking into* TIRI's
> *house and raping her. The braying horns are louder. In a*
> *rage,* TILLY *returns* TIRI's *attack and, this time, it is* TIRI
> *who is on the retreat.*

TILLY (*to* TIRI): You wouldn't leave it alone, would you.

TIRI: You should never have let them do that to you.

TILLY: Oh? And how was I supposed to stop them?

TIRI: You should have fought to stop them from entering you.

> *The peruperu duel now escalates.* TILLY's *strength is*
> *pitted against* TIRI's *cunning, as* TIRI *uses her wheelchair*
> *to defend against close-quarters attack. Eventually, how-*
> *ever,* TILLY *gains the upper hand and sends* TIRI's
> *wheelchair spinning away.* TIRI *throws her peruperu staff*
> *to one side favouring, instead, her two walking sticks as*
> *weapons.*

TILLY: There were four of them —

TIRI: The numbers don't matter. Because they had their way.
    And they planted their seed in you.

> TILLY *sweeps* TIRI's *walking sticks away from her and*
> TIRI *falls to the floor. She puts up a hand to* TILLY.

TIRI: You wouldn't hit a poor defenceless woman when she's
    lying on the ground, would you?

> TILLY *hesitates.* TIRI *mimes throwing dust in her eyes,*
> *and* TILLY *staggers back, momentarily blinded.* TIRI

> *manages to sit up, but with a scream of anger,* TILLY *has pushed her back down again, jabbing at her while she is lying on the floor.* TIRI *turns one way to escape the first jab and another way to escape the second jab. But it is no use.* TILLY *puts the point of her peruperu stick at* TIRI's *throat.*

TILLY: Had enough, old lady?

> TILLY *turns her back on* TIRI *and begins to walk away. With a hiss,* TIRI *stands on her walking sticks and, with a swiftness that is surprising, pursues* TILLY. *At the last moment,* TIRI *throws her walking sticks away and, using the momentum of her body, throws herself at* TILLY. *They sway together, locked in each other's grasp.* TILLY *realises that* TIRI *is spiralling again. The horns are at their loudest.*

TILLY: Enough, Tiri. Enough!

> *The horns suddenly stop. In the dramatic silence,* TIRI *looks at* TILLY *and gives her a knife. The moon comes up.*

TIRI (*shouting*): You should have killed it.

TILLY: I couldn't.

TIRI: When Pirimia was born, you should have – killed –

> TIRI *is shaking apart.* TILLY *puts the knife back in* TIRI's *hands.* TIRI *sways, looking at the knife.* TILLY *finally reveals herself as* TIRI's *conscience by forcing her to face up to the secret of Pirimia.*

TILLY (*in a gentle voice*): Kill your own son?

TIRI: The smell of a newborn child —

TILLY (*forgivingly*): Satan's spawn? Pale? With eyes at the back of his head?

TIRI: The feel of one's own flesh against your skin —

TILLY (*forcefully*): He brings death. Kill him.

> *On the soundtrack a baby wails. With a sob,* TIRI *drops the knife. It clatters to the floor. And, suddenly, the two women are holding each other tightly.*

TIRI: I should never have left those old weavers.

TILLY: You should not blame yourself for being a twelve-year-old girl.

TIRI: When those men did that to me, I should have fought harder. Harder.

TILLY: Forgive yourself, Kui. There is always a reason for everything.

> *It is a struggle for* TIRI *to acknowledge this.*

Scene Five

On the soundtrack we hear the rustling sounds of a huge bird flying into the auditorium.

TILLY: Ah well, darling, one more public appearance. The

governor-general's here. Your telegram has arrived.

TIRI: Do we have to?

TILLY: Yes.

> *On the soundtrack the sound of clapping.*

FRED (*V/O*): This way, your excellency.

> TIRI *and* TILLY, *onstage, are staring ahead at the audience. They are chanting the following, using the appropriate hand and facial actions.*

TIRI/TILLY: Nō wai te motokā e topa mai na i te rori?
>> Auē! Nāu e kawana-tianara, kei te haere tika mai ki ahau!
>> Whose is the car speeding along the highway?
>> It is yours, governor-general, coming straight at me –
>> Auē hi! Auē hi! Auē ha! Auē hi! Auē hi! Auē ha!

> TIRI *and* TILLY *have stilled – but their hands are shivering in the very dramatic movement of the wiri and their eyes are wide in the pūkana.*

GOVERNOR-GENERAL (*V/O*): It is my honour, Mrs Mahana, on the occasion of your 160th birthday, to offer you Her Royal Highness Queen Elizabeth's birthday greetings. You are the oldest woman in the Commonwealth and, indeed, the world. Her majesty offers you her warmest wishes on this auspicious occasion.

> *During the foregoing* TILLY *is performing movements associated with the wero. She approaches the audience and bends down and mimes receiving the telegram. She takes the telegram back to* TIRI. *Flashbulbs are popping, flash, flash, flash. Then* TILLY's *attention is taken by a rain of silver dust.*

TILLY: Hey! Guess who's here!

> TIRI *gives an indrawn cry – of fear, but then of acceptance. She closes her eyes and relaxes. She begins to remonstrate, waving her walking sticks angrily at Death.*

TIRI (*angrily*): Kei whea koe? I kōrero ahau ki a koe, kia hoki mai i te toru tekau tau! Where have you been? I told you to come back in thirty years! You should be fired! (*Suddenly,* TIRI *gasps and turns to talk to somebody else.*) Is that you, Mum? Is it time to go home now?

> *Tenderly,* TILLY *approaches* TIRI. TIRI *looks up at her, a glow of excitement on her face.*

TIRI: Has Mum come to get me?

TILLY: Āe.

> TIRI *sighs with contentment. She leans back in* TILLY's *arms, as if in the arms of a lover. Then her eyes snap open.*

TIRI: Hang on a moment.

> *But* TILLY *is returning to the 'doorway' position on the set. She begins wrapping herself in her dreams, her arms outstretched to* TIRI.
> TIRI *picks up the telegram. She looks at the audience. She spits on the telegram. But she still hesitates. She wants to go but –*
> TIRI *looks up into the auditorium.*

TIRI: Jessica, whakarongo –

JESSICA (*V/O*): Please don't go, Nani, please don't leave me all alone, please –

> JESSICA *begins to sob and moan.* TIRI *levers herself up from the wheelchair and walks on her sticks to the very front of the stage.*

TIRI (*brokenly*): Kaua koe e tangi, moko –

> *But* JESSICA *continues to sob.* TIRI *becomes reproving and stern. She has been fighting all her life. She stamps her walking sticks for* JESSICA's *attention.*

Hope! Ringa whiua! Ka panapana –
Moko! Whakarongo! Ka panapana –
I a ha ha! Ka rekareka tonu taku ngākau pōhatu whakapiri –

> TIRI *pauses, listening. Gradually* JESSICA's *sobs subside.*

JESSICA (*V/O, in a faltering voice*): Kia haere mai!
Te takitini!
Kia haere mai –

*JESSICA's voice sounds as if it is coming out of the future.
Her voice is joined by other young children's voices.*

JESSICA/OTHERS (*V/O*): Te takimano kia pare tai tokotia ki
        Aotearoa!
    Hi ha auē!
    He mamae, he mamae —

TIRI *listens to the voices, her face expressionless and eternal.*

END

Huia Playscripts

Willie Craig Fransen	*Taku Waimarie*
Briar Grace-Smith	*Ngā Pou Wāhine*
	Purapurawhetū
Witi Ihimaera	*Woman Far Walking*
Hone Kouka	*Waiora*